PRESENT KNOWLEDGE IN NUTRITION

PREPARED FROM ARTICLES
WRITTEN ESPECIALLY FOR

NUTRITION REVIEWS
on the

TWENTY-FIFTH ANNIVERSARY
of the

NUTRITION FOUNDATION

PUBLISHED BY

THE NUTRITION FOUNDATION, INC.
NINETY-NINE PARK AVENUE • NEW YORK, N.Y. 10016

CONTENTS

CHAPTER I

PRESENT KNOWLEDGE OF CALORIES

OGDEN C. JOHNSON, PH.D.

Much early work in nutrition was devoted to the study of calories, or more correctly, energy metabolism. By the late 1920's, excellent reviews on this subject were being published. Research scientists in the 1930's and 1940's worked out rather precise values for the energy requirements of man under varying conditions. Five or six basic areas have been investigated in relation to the total energy requirement of man.

Basal metabolism, which accounts for the largest quantity of energy expenditure, has usually been related to body surface. Many articles have been published attempting to establish normal values for basal metabolism. When basal metabolic rate is expressed on the basis of surface area, or any formula which takes total size into consideration, there is relatively small variation between individuals of the same sex and age. In recent years, more consideration has been given to those factors which tend to modify the basal metabolic rate. It has been established that the metabolic rate decreases as one grows older. In establishing caloric requirements, this decrease in metabolic rate is generally taken into consideration. In addition, it has been found that metabolic rate increases during pregnancy, thus accounting for part of the increase of caloric demand which is associated with this condition. This increase during pregnancy may be as much as 20 per cent over the basal metabolic rate found prior to pregnancy.

Studies on the effects of starvation have indicated that there is a reduction in basal metabolic rate after periods of two or three weeks of starvation or severe caloric restriction. Studies by A. Keys and co-workers have indicated that prolonged starvation can result in a reduction of basal metabolic rate to less than 50 per cent of the prestarvation rate. This reduction appears to be an adaptation which enables the body to conserve energy (F. Grande, J. P. Anderson, H. L. Taylor, and Keys, *Fed. Proc.* **16,** *49* (*1957*)).

Body composition also has some effect on metabolic rate although this is not of the magnitude related to starvation. Individuals with large muscular development have a basal metabolic rate from 5 to 6 per cent greater than that of persons of the same height and weight, but with less muscle mass. Some consideration has been given to utilizing the relationship of basal metabolic rate to body composition as a parameter of comparison. However, the difficulties in obtaining accurate measurements of body composition make this method, although theoretically more exact, considerably more difficult than comparison to body surface. While the collection of data on factors affecting basal metabolic rate, particularly diseases which affect the secretion of ductless glands and certain drugs, has continued, there has been relatively little new basic information developed in recent years in this area of energy metabolism.

Energy expenditure related to activity is the second largest component of caloric expenditure in man. Studies on the caloric expenditure associated with various types of work have illustrated that it is difficult to greatly increase total energy expenditure by activity, except for brief periods. Many tables have been published giving caloric expenditure values for various activities. The basic caloric costs for activities will be related to the caloric costs of the activity as influenced by the body size of the individual and will be directly related to the length of time spent carrying out the activity. The effect of body size has been carefully studied, and it is apparent that larger individuals will utilize more energy in performing a given activity than a smaller person (M. S. Malhotra, S. S. Ramaswamy, and S. N. Roy, *J. Appl. Physiol.* **17**, *433* (*1962*)).

In general, the caloric requirements of complicated and difficult tasks play a small part in the total daily caloric expenditure of the average individual. Of more concern are the caloric costs of the normal activities, such as walking, standing, sitting, eating, dressing, and undressing. Individuals living a rather sedentary life will probably carry out few tasks which have a caloric cost as great as 3.5 calories per hour per kilogram of body weight. Tasks requiring this magnitude of caloric expenditure or greater constitute hard physical labor, particularly for individuals who are normally sedentary.

The amount of time which must be put into a task such as walking, in order to consume a significant amount of energy, illustrates quite clearly why most physical activity does not in itself lead to marked reductions in body weight of obese individuals. An individual sitting utilizes approximately 0.5 calories per kilogram per hour. Walking at a moderate speed for a period of one hour would only slightly more than double the caloric expenditure. Most individuals find an hour's walk a rather unrewarding task in relation to the calories consumed. In general, increasing caloric expenditure by exercise, although potentially of great importance in equalizing caloric intake and output, does not serve in this manner in the sedentary individual who over a decade gains from five to ten pounds and after a 25 or 30 year period finds himself from 20 to 30 pounds over the desirable weight for his height and age.

No factor associated with energy metabolism has been less understood than the *specific dynamic effect*, and though the rise in heat production associated with the ingestion of food was pointed out over 50 years ago, exact determination of the factors that cause this effect has not yet been worked out. It is apparent, however, that a small amount of the energy consumed as food is utilized in the production of heat, and this energy, designated as *specific dynamic effect*, is directly related to the food ingested. It has been demonstrated that one cannot add *specific dynamic effect* of individual foods, but that it is necessary to establish the *specific dynamic effect* of the total diet.

Only about 6 per cent of the energy intake is consumed by specific dynamic effect; thus it is not of major consideration in establishing caloric requirements. The apparent waste of energy due to this effect has been given considerable thought, since it does not conform to the concepts of energy conservation frequently attributed to the human organism.

Many other factors also affect energy metabolism; among these are the temperatures in which the person is living. It has been generally assumed that man's caloric requirements increase at very low temperatures, but this is less important when adequate clothing is worn. Since heat production is related to the regulation of body temperature, some control must be available in order to maintain desirable body temperature. In elevated temperatures, normal body temperature is achieved by the evaporation of water from the skin and lungs. There is evidence that the caloric requirement at extremely high temperatures is slightly increased due to the energy required to transfer water to the surface to achieve sweating and to maintain body temperature.

Consideration is given to temperature in the calculation of caloric requirements. This factor, however, is of minor significance in terms of individuals existing in climates where temperature variation is small. More consideration should be given to this problem, however, in zones where temperature differences at various times of the year may be as much as 50 or 60°F., and where protection from the environment is less complete than in the United States.

While information on some aspects of energy requirements and caloric expenditure appears to be complete, questions on specific dynamic effect, caloric requirement for weight maintenance in obese individuals, and the relationship of body composition to calorie sources have not been satisfactorily answered. Thus, even after many years of careful study, statements on caloric requirements, sources of calories and energy, and relationship of the composition of the diet to the availability of energy must be carefully qualified. An example of this was found in the report of D. S. Miller and P. R. Payne (*J. Nutrition* **78**, *255* (*1962*)), which suggested that under certain conditions animals can maintain a body weight on caloric intakes which vary widely. Their study on pigs raised many questions which have not been satisfactorily answered, such as:

Can food energy be converted directly to heat energy? Under certain conditions, can an animal metabolize all food eaten? These are among a few of the questions which need to be answered, before it can be said that energy metabolism and energy requirements are understood.

One of the practical aspects of energy is expressed in the development of caloric requirements for various population groups. The original report of the Committee on Calorie Requirements of the Food and Agriculture Organization (FAO) of the United Nations appeared in 1950. Since that time, there has been a continuing reassessment by nutritionists of the caloric requirements under various physiological situations. The second FAO report on calories, developed in 1957, continued in the same general direction as the first committee, using the "Reference Standard" but adding certain modifications to answer some of the criticisms which had been made of the first report.

Basic to the concept of establishing "Caloric Requirements" is the development of a reference standard. In both FAO reports, the reference man is 25 years of age, weighs 65 kg., lives in a temperate zone with a mean annual temperature of 10°C., maintains his weight, and has a work program that keeps him active for eight hours each day. He is sedentary four hours each day and sleeps about eight hours each day. About one and one-half hours are spent in recreation or household work, and about one and one-half hours walking. This man is said to require 3,200 calories daily.

The reference woman is described in a similar manner, her weight is 55 kg., her age 25 years, and she maintains a home. Her caloric requirement in assumed to be 2,300 calories. Pregnancy and lactation can alter the basic caloric requirement of the reference woman. The increased caloric need associated with pregnancy is the balance between reduced activity as the result of the pregnancy, and the caloric demands imposed by the increase of basal metabolic rate of the pregnant woman, and the growing fetus. A recommended allowance of 40,000 calories per pregnancy is said to cover the net increase in caloric requirement.

The caloric cost of lactation in terms of milk has been carefully studied in many laboratories, but less is known about the efficiency of production and caloric cost in addition to that of the milk. The FAO committee indicated that 1,000 calories per day would be a satisfactory allowance for lactation.

The question, always asked concerning nutritional allowances, is how were the values determined. It is apparent that many assumptions must be made even to start to establish a reference standard. Since FAO requirement values are to be used in many countries, it is well to consider the factors which must be included.

One of the most important factors is height and weight. In most countries of the world, height and weight is significantly less than that of the developed nations such as the United States and those of Western Europe. While questions as to the health hazards of obesity have been used to suggest that larger physical size can be detrimental to health, it is apparent that healthy individuals with long life spans are found in the developed countries. The compromise figure of 65 kg. for the reference man is less than that selected by the Food and Nutrition Board of the National Academy of Sciences-National Research Council (*Recommended Dietary Allowances, Sixth Revised Edition. Washington, D.C., 1964*), but more than the average weight in many countries. For calculation of caloric requirements using the FAO standards, it is better to use the actual mean weight for the population within a country and the caloric requirement calculated on a per kilogram basis. Tables have been included in the FAO report giving average male caloric requirements for other weights ranging from 45 to 80 kg.

Once the height and weight figures are established, it is necessary to select an activity profile and the type of environment. For international tables, figures must be selected to give the widest use to the basic tables of caloric requirements. To be meaningful, caloric requirements for a country should be based on actual weight and activity.

The 1964 revision of the *Recommended Dietary Allowances* made several changes in relation to caloric requirements. In the past, the energy expenditure of the "reference" man has been considered to be moderate, with only short periods of high energy expenditure. With the continued increase in mean body weight in the United States, it is apparent that the actual caloric intakes have been greater than total expenditure. For this reason, the 1964 *Recommended Dietary Allowances* has reduced caloric

allowances for the "reference" man and woman from 3,200 and 2,300 to 2,900 and 2,100 calories respectively.

In addition, the 1964 revision has recognized the reduced energy requirements as a person grows older. While part of this decrease is associated with a reduced basal metabolic rate as one becomes older, a portion of the reduced requirement in the United States population is related to reduced physical activity. Increasing body weight with age, observed in the United States population, is not seen in many other countries, particularly those in some of the developing areas of the world. Animal experiments suggest that longevity is often associated with slight under-nutrition. The data from insurance companies indicate that in some cases the weight gain associated with increasing age is related to higher mortality and morbidity. The correction for age reduces the caloric allowance for the 70 kg. "reference" man from 2,900 calories at age 25 to 2,200 calories at age 65.

In recent years, considerably more interest has developed in the actual energy production in muscles and in other tissues. Since the early 1900's, it has been known that muscle work results in the production of lactic acid, and that the lactic acid comes from glycogen in the muscle. In 1930, contraction was produced in muscles poisoned with iodoacetate without the formation of lactic acid, suggesting that some other source of energy was also available to the muscle. Further research indicated that phosphocreatine could serve as a source of energy for muscle. Other studies established that certain high energy compounds such as adenosinetriphosphate (ATP) were involved as an energy source in muscle contraction (D. R. Cain and R. E. Davies, *Biochem. Biophys. Res. Commun.* **8**, *361* (*1962*)).

While the immediate source of energy for work is high energy compounds, production of these compounds from food calories must be considered. For many years it was assumed that only carbohydrate could be used as a source of energy for muscular work. Thus glucose or its precursors have been considered the most important components in the diet for muscle work. In recent years it has been established that muscles can also utilize fatty acids as a source of energy (S. J. Friedberg, W. R. Horlan, Jr., D. L. Trout, and H. H. Estes, Jr., *J. Clin. Invest.* **39,** *215* (*1960*); R. J. Havel, A. Naimark, and C. H. Borchgrevink, *Ibid.* **42,** *1054* (*1963*)). These fatty acids are primarily derived from adipose tissue; however, a large portion of this tissue is probably originally derived from dietary carbohydrate.

The relationship of the two basic calorie sources for muscle work has not been clearly determined, but it is apparent that free fatty acid levels in the blood are controlled by various hormones, and this hormonal control may be related to physical fitness. Studies on trained men have shown that plasma free fatty acid levels are higher and turnover rate is increased as compared with sedentary man (L. A. Cobb and W. P. Johnson, *J. Clin. Invest.* **42,** *800* (*1963*)). At the present time there is considerable interest in this aspect of energy intake among athletes and coaches. More work is needed in this area before consideration can be given to feeding specific diets to improve performance.

While many of the basic questions concerning calories were answered from 20 to 50 years ago, the most practical aspect of calories and energy remains one of our major health problems. With an estimated 40,000,000 people in the United States classified as obese, or at least overweight, it is not surprising that discussions of calories and diets rank near the top of current topics at cocktail parties and women's clubs. Though the scientific information on calories is known, it appears that we have not been able to convince man that these facts hold the answer to the problem of obesity.

Calories are calories, yet each month one finds a new diet, supported with a veneer of scientific information, offered to the public. The "low carbohydrate" and "high fat" diets claim to overcome the problem of calories. The lack of scientific support for these diets has been reviewed by R. E. Hodges (*Nutrition Reviews* **24,** *65* (*1966*)). It is apparent that not one of these diets is really successful. If it were, there would be no need for the continuing stream of diets and fads.

The reduction in energy expenditure because of automation in the United States probably is responsible for part of the increasing incidence of obesity. Of equal importance, however, may be the increasing supply of high calorie food items, and the ability of most persons to purchase these foods. Basic scientific information on calories and energy will not give sufficient answers for the problems of excess caloric intake. The individual *willing* and *able* to match caloric intake and output can solve this health problem.

Chapter II

PRESENT KNOWLEDGE OF PROTEIN NUTRITION

W. Duane Brown, Ph.D.

The primary function of proteins in diets is to supply amino acids. Of the 20 or so amino acids utilized in the synthesis of proteins, eight must be supplied in the diet of man. Biosynthesis of the others requires a dietary nitrogen source, which is ordinarily protein. However, mixtures of amino acids in the proper proportion will support animal life. Such mixtures may be less well utilized than intact proteins (Q. R. Rogers and A. E. Harper, *J. Nutrition* **87,** *267* (*1965*); W. D. Salmon, *Ibid.* **82,** *76* (*1964*); R. A. Ahrens, J. E. Wilson, and M. Womack, *Ibid.* **88,** *219* (*1966*)). Measurements of nitrogen balance, *i.e.*, the difference between intake and output, are useful, but values obtained represent only an algebraic sum of gains and losses.

The digestion of proteins is to some extent self-controlling, in that ingestion of proteins stimulates production or release of hydrochloric acid and proteolytic enzymes in the gastrointestinal tract. For example, an increase in the level of dietary protein results in an increased release of pancreatic proteases (J. T. Snook, *J. Nutrition* **87,** *297* (*1965*)). The pancreatic enzymes released to the intestine provide a substantial portion of the so-called endogenous protein. Such protein, together with that from turnover of mucosal membrane cells, is considered by some to provide efficiency in absorption and utilization and to prevent large fluctuations in the assortment of amino acids available for absorption (*Nutrition Reviews* **20,** *79* (*1962*); E. S. Nasset, *Fed. Proc.* **24,** *953* (*1965*)). This reasonable hypothesis is not in line with the fact that the removal of one or more essential amino acids from the diet of animals results in an almost immediate negative response.

In adult animals, only amino acids are absorbed, there being no appreciable transfer of intact proteins across the intestinal wall. Amino acids are absorbed at different rates (*Nutrition Reviews* **20,** *306* (*1962*); **21,** *97* (*1963*)). However, rate of absorption is not synonymous with nutritional superiority. Proteins of high biological value are absorbed not too rapidly (W. H. Griffith, *Am. J. Clin. Nutrition* **17,** *391* (*1965*)), possibly providing for more uniform release of amino acids and less waste.

A biochemical explanation for the process of absorption is not yet possible. F. Alvarado (*Science* **151,** *1010* (*1966*)) has suggested that there is a sodium ion-dependent membrane carrier, protein in nature, which has separate binding sites for sugars, neutral amino acids, basic amino acids, and sodium ion. The transfer of amino acids between plasma and cells is a process closely related to the transfer of amino acids from the intestine to the plasma. It is generally assumed that the mechanisms involved are similar.

This transfer is an uphill phenomenon, there being many times the concentration of amino acids in tissues as in plasma. Measurements of cellular amino acid nitrogen at varying time intervals following exposure to plasma amino acids show that amino acids are not immediately metabolized or incorporated into cellular structures, but are taken into the cells as free amino acids. The accumulated amino acids provide homeostasis and allow, within limits, intermittent feeding. This homeostatic capacity is limited, since excess protein in the diet is promptly metabolized.

Cellular uptake of amino acids depends upon their distribution between plasma and cell. H. N. Christensen (*Fed. Proc.* **22,** *1110* (*1963*)) called attention to the fact that one must consider both plasma and tissue level of amino acids in relation to each other. It is well established that there is competition for transport sites (*Nutrition Reviews* **21,** *97* (*1963*)). Some evidence indicates that within the group of neutral amino acids there exist two transfer sites, one for the transport of straight chain neutral amino acids and one for the transport of branched chain amino acids.

Removal of any essential amino acid from the diet will result in a general lowering of protein synthesis and increased nitrogen excretion. Some proteins present in the animal organism may, however, respond to a dietary inadequacy by at least a transient increase in synthetic rates. Thus, it has been demonstrated that threonine deficient diets given rats may enhance the incorporation of amino acids into selected proteins (*Nutrition Reviews* **23,** *111* (*1965*)).

Obviously, such enhanced synthesis could not continue indefinitely. The increase in synthesis of certain proteins under the stress of a dietary deficiency of amino acids may afford a measure of protection. Caloric intake has a substantial influence on protein synthesis, in that caloric restriction results in a substantial increase in nitrogen excretion due to the utilization of tissue proteins for energy. Conversely, addition of carbohydrate or fat to calorically inadequate diets produces increased nitrogen retention.

Insulin and other hormones have significant effects on protein metabolism. Generally, adrenal corticoids and thyroid are catabolic, and influence the transfer of muscle protein, through the plasma amino acid pool, to liver for metabolism and elimination, while other hormones, including insulin, growth hormone, and testosterone, are anabolic in nature, resulting in a buildup of muscle proteins. Insulin stimulates protein synthesis in muscle and induces a decrease in the concentration of plasma amino acids. These effects apparently are due to both an influence on amino acid transport and a stimulation of protein synthesis at sites distal to transport (I. G. Wool, *Fed. Proc.* **24,** *1060* (*1965*)).

Recent evidence (*Nutrition Reviews* **23,** *125* (*1965*)) suggests that dietary ethionine inhibits protein synthesis by combining with adenosinetriphosphate (ATP), removing it as an energy source and inhibiting the production of messenger ribonucleic acid (RNA). The effect of vitamin D on calcium transport may be due to its involvement in the synthesis of a protein carried (*Ibid.* **24,** *18* (*1966*)). Vitamin E deficient rabbits have been shown to incorporate more labeled amino acids into mucle protein than controls. However, this effect seems to be due to a higher uptake into the amino acid pool, rather than an increase in protein synthesis per se. The increased uptake may be due to alterations of cell permeability in vitamin E deficient animals (J. F. Diehl, *Nature* **209,** *75* (*1966*)).

The effect of ethanol on liver lipid accumulation has been ascribed to blockage of lipoprotein synthesis. However, animals given ethanol incorporate labeled amino acids into hepatic proteins at approximately the same rate as controls (*Nutrition Reviews* **24,** *21* (*1966*)).

Efforts to define minimum requirements for protein are limited by the adequacy of criteria used. Studies of protein requirements are conducted usually by one of three approaches: (1) determination of the amount of an essential amino acid required to maintain nitrogen balance in subjects receiving an otherwise adequate diet; (2) determination of the amount of protein required to maintain nitrogen balance; and (3) estimation of obligatory losses of nitrogen that must be replaced by dietary protein. An expert group of FAO-WHO has used the third approach to estimate requirements of man (*WHO Technical Report Series, No. 301. Geneva, 1965*). They recommend an intake of 0.59 g. protein per kilogram body weight per day for an average adult; 0.88 g. for a one to three year old child; and 2.3 g. for a newborn to three months old infant. These are practical recommendations for the so-called average man. All values are for a "reference" protein considered to be fully utilized; it is necessary to correct such values for the quality of protein actually used. In spite of some justified criticism leveled at these recommendations (E. G. Holmes, *World Rev. Nutrition Dietet.* **5**, *237* (*1965*)), they likely represent as good an estimate as is currently available.

A variety of factors may influence requirements. The FAO report does not consider any change with age once adulthood is reached. There is some indication, however, that requirements may be increased in older subjects (R. W. Wannemacher, Jr., and J. R. McCoy, *J. Nutrition* **88**, *66* (*1966*); S. G. Tuttle *et al., Am. J. Clin. Nutrition* **16**, *225* (*1955*); *Ibid.* **16**, *229* (*1955*)).

Requirements for protein may be influenced by caloric intake. On a fixed adequate protein intake the energy level of the diet will determine nitrogen balance, while on a fixed caloric intake the protein level is the determining factor (D. H. Calloway and H. Spector, *Am. J. Clin. Nutrition* **2**, *405* (*1954*)). Proteins ordinarily are not used for energy when adequate carbohydrate and fat calories are available, but at caloric intakes below the needs of an animal, available protein is metabolized.

The stress of cold may cause a temporary increase in nitrogen excretion with a resulting increase in requirement (*Nutrition Reviews* **21**, *78* (*1963*)); long-term studies need to be undertaken.

An additional allowance of protein during pregnancy is probably not necessary for women who normally consume liberal quantities of protein. The FAO group, estimating that 950 g. of protein are utilized for maternal tissue and fetal growth, suggests an additional requirement of reference protein of 6 g. per day during the last two trimesters. They also estimate an increased requirement of 30 g. per day of protein at the upper limit of lactation.

Protein requirement must be considered in relation to protein quality. The quality of a protein depends upon its proportions of amino acids. A "balanced" protein contains amino acids in good proportion relative to the amounts required by an animal. Other than the amino acid content, the main factor influencing quality is digestibility.

There is little agreement on the best way experimentally to determine protein quality. Most techniques are based on growth response, nitrogen balance, or amino acid concentrations. A summary of terms and formulas used in protein quality evaluation has appeared in a useful publication (*National Academy of Sciences-National Research Council, publication 1100. Washington, D.C., 1963*). Two traditional methods remain popular, namely, Biological Value and Protein Efficiency Ratio. The former measures retention of absorbed nitrogen; a modification of it, the Net Protein Utilization, measures retention of nitrogen based on intake rather than that absorbed.

Both are based upon differences in carcass nitrogen between the test group and a group fed no protein. Because of the relationship between carcass water content and nitrogen content there has been a tendency to use the simpler determination of water content in such assays (*Nutrition Reviews* **20**, *319* (*1962*)). The Protein Efficiency Ratio (weight gain per weight of protein eaten) is less laborious, since only growth need be measured, but a straight line function often is not obtained. Many techniques use nitrogen balance measurements and frequently are based upon the relationship between nitrogen balance and absorbed nitrogen (Nitrogen Balance Index). None of these methods is particularly well suited for use with human beings. Efforts to use the levels of plasma amino acids have been made (*Ibid.* **21**, *138* (*1963*); J. M. McLaughlin, *Fed. Proc.* **22**, *1122* (*1963*)).

Generally, animal proteins are of better quality than vegetable. Cereal proteins are often low in lysine and in some cases methionine and/or tryptophan; pulses may be low in methionine, and oil seeds and nuts are often deficient in lysine and methionine. C. V. Kies, E. Williams, and H. M. Fox (*J. Nutrition* **86**, *350* (*1965*)) suggest that nonspecific nitrogen, *i.e.*, nonessential rather than tryptophan, is the first limiting factor in corn protein. That cottonseed protein is limiting in lysine and methionine has been questioned by H. Fisher (*Ibid.* **87**, *9* (*1965*)), who concludes that threonine, leucine, and isoleucine are also limiting.

Genetic factors can have significant influences on protein quality. An excellent example of this is the recent development of corn having higher concentrations of lysine and tryptophan (*Nutrition Reviews* **23**, *336* (*1965*); W. M. Beeson *et al.*, *Foodstuffs* **38**, *7* (*1966*)). The quality of protein found in this strain of corn is improved over that in ordinary corn and its nutritional adequacy has been demonstrated. High protein diets are probably not deleterious. Ingestion of large quantities of protein usually results in increased excretion. Activities of the urea cycle enzymes, measured in liver homogenates, are markedly increased in animals on high protein diets. Such findings have been corroborated by an *in vivo* study with rats (*Nutrition Reviews* **22**, *280* (*1964*)).

The term "amino acid imbalance" generally refers to a pattern of amino acids in the diet that induces a growth depression which can be overcome by supplementation with the most limiting amino acid or acids. For example, growth and food intake are depressed in rats fed a low protein diet containing an excess of an essential amino acid (A. E. Harper, R. V. Becker, and W. P. Stucki, *Proc. Soc. Exp. Biol. Med.* **121**, *695* (*1966*)). At least part of the effect of such imbalances is due to an influence on food consumption (J. C. Sanahuja and Harper, *Am. J. Physiol.* **202**, *165* (*1962*); Sanahuja, M. E. Rio, and M. N. Lede, *J. Nutrition* **86**, *424* (*1965*)).

The term "amino acid antagonism" ordinarily refers to a pattern of amino acids in diets that causes growth depression which can be overcome by supplementation with an amino acid structurally similar to the antagonist. In contrast to imbalance, the supplemented amino acids need not be limiting. For example, the addition of excess lysine to the diet of chicks depressed growth and caused symptoms similar to those seen in arginine deficient chickens; addition of small amounts of arginine to the diet reversed the adverse effects (*Nutrition Reviews* **23**, *139* (*1965*)). One result of imbalance or antagonism is an increase in the requirement for an amino acid present in amounts that would otherwise be adequate.

The term "amino acid toxicity" is applied to a situation in which the adverse effect cannot be overcome by supplementation. Thus, methionine fed in excessive amounts to rats caused a marked inhibition of growth and depression of food intake with associated pathological changes; these effects could not be overcome by a variety of supplements (*Nutrition Reviews* **23**, *202* (*1965*)). The effects described above are not usually seen in human populations.

For man, the most important changes in malnutrition are those due to insufficient intake of protein or intake of protein of poor quality. While there are no storage depots for protein similar to those for fat and carbohydrates, such stores as are available (reserves) may be important as a defense against short-term protein deprivation. Some tissue proteins are depleted rapidly when animals are placed on protein free diets, and such animals have increased efficiency in retaining dietary nitrogen (J. B. Allison and Wannemacher, *Am. J. Clin. Nutrition* **16**, *445* (*1965*)).

Continued inadequacy of dietary protein causes serious effects on tissue proteins. Plasma proteins change, albumins particularly being substantially reduced. There may be a decrease in synthesis of albumin but no decrease in synthesis of gamma-globulins in children with kwashiorkor (*Nutrition Reviews* **21**, *172, 209* (*1963*)). The lowering of hemoglobin levels in states of protein insufficiency is generally ascribed to a lack of amino acids necessary for synthesizing the protein. However, in protein deficient animals there is also reduced production of erythropoietin (*Ibid.* **23**, *242* (*1965*)). Body proteins other than those in the blood and liver are also affected, *e.g.*, those present in bone (*Ibid.* **21**, *242* (*1963*)).

The edema associated with protein malnutrition is attributed to a variety of factors including alterations in osmotic pressure caused by changes in protein concentration. There is a marked decrease in extracellular fluid volume (*Nutrition Reviews* **24**, *75* (*1966*)).

As a result of protein deprivation there is a marked depression in levels of vitamin A in plasma, presumably associated with a lack of transport protein. Other vitamins are relatively unaffected. There are many changes in enzyme activities accompanying protein deficiency, including a reduction in the level of urea cycle enzymes and an accompanying reduction in urea excretion (*Nutrition Reviews* **21**, *54* (*1963*)). Most liver enzymes show a decline in activity, but the levels of some are unchanged and a few may increase (*Ibid.* **20**, *280* (*1962*)).

Rats deprived of protein show a substantial increase in activity of liver amino acid activating enzymes (*Nutrition Reviews* **21**, *344* (*1963*)), a phenomenon

probably associated with a survival mechanism. It is hoped that certain of these changes may some day be utilized to diagnose preclinical kwashiorkor. In this connection it is significant that workers have been able to develop a kwashiorkor-like syndrome in rats (*Ibid.* **23**, *27* (*1965*)) and in pigs (*Ibid.* **25**, *205* (*1965*)).

Of the various anomalies of amino acid absorption and metabolism, phenylketonuria has attracted the most attention. The condition results in mental aberrations in infants. Those affected have a block in the conversion of phenylalanine to tyrosine, with the resulting accumulation of high serum levels of phenylalanine and the excretion of excessive amounts of certain of its metabolites. Animals in which the disorder is induced have reduced learning ability (*Nutrition Reviews* **22**, *124* (*1964*)). The reason for brain damage is not known.

Other anomalies include homocystinuria, caused by absence of cystathionine synthetase; cystathioninuria; and alcaptonuria. The latter results from the absence of homogentisic acid oxidase, causing an accumulation of homogentisic acid which may deposit, in polymeric form, in connective tissue.

Maple sugar urine disease (named for the odor) is due to a block in the oxidative decarboxylation of branched chain amino acids. These materials accumulate in the blood and are excreted in large amounts in urine. Early dietary regulation may result in some amelioration of the disease, which is ordinarily fatal (*Nutrition Reviews* **23**, *260* (*1965*)).

Among other aminoacidurias reported are those involving citrulline and alloisoleucine (*Nutrition Reviews* **20**, *197* (*1962*)), and several involving a defect in absorption and transport (*see* S. J. Saunders and K. J. Isselbacher, *Gastroenterology* **50**, *586* (*1966*); *Nutrition Reviews* **22**, *138* (*1964*)).

Within the United States there probably is no significant problem of dietary inadequacy of protein. However, severe problems do exist in many parts of the world. The prevalence of kwashiorkor has been the object of considerable study, and many efforts have been made to relieve this problem. Approaches suggested include better utilization of available vegetable proteins, supplementation of diets with protein concentrates or amino acids, and increasing the amount of animal proteins in diets. A few of these programs, such as those using Incaparina and the Indian multi-purpose food have had some success. The recent approval of the U.S. Food and Drug Administration (*see the Federal Register, February 2, 1967*) of limited commercial production of whole fish protein concentrate will allow utilization of an important new resource. Such concentrates, with high levels of excellent quality protein, could prove to be a major factor in the alleviation of protein malnutrition throughout the world. Ultimate solutions are not now limited by inadequacy of knowledge of protein nutrition, but rather by technological and sociological considerations.

CHAPTER III

PRESENT KNOWLEDGE OF CARBOHYDRATES

ROBERT E. HODGES, M.D.

Carbohydrates comprise the most varied and plentiful foods in the world. Because they give the highest yield of energy per acre of land they may be considered among the most important to human survival. The populations of the world derive more than half of their nutrients from carbohydrate foods, which vary from one part of the world to another but share the same things in common. They are relatively easy to grow, and hence inexpensive; highly palatable, and can be stored for reasonable periods of time without undue deterioration. Classic examples of these staple foods include rice, corn, wheat, and potatoes.

Fortunately, like most carbohydrates from natural sources, these foods carry with them substantial quantities of important vitamins and minerals in addition to small but valuable amounts of protein. Although vegetable proteins, in general, have a lower biological value—i.e., an amino acid mixture which is less ideal for mammalian growth—than animal protein, they still make a vital contribution to the total protein content of the diet. It probably is no accident that in most nations there is at least one traditional and favorite recipe combining vegetable or grain products with milk or cheese or other animal foods, a mixture which greatly enhances both the amino acid pattern and the flavor. For example, in oriental countries rice frequently is served with small quantities of fish or meat.

Housewives throughout the world would have great difficulty in preparing attractive meals if foods containing carbohydrate became scarce. Every race of people has welcomed the carbohydrate foods, including even the Eskimos, who have a fondness for breads and sweets whenever they can be obtained (P. Freuchen, *Book of the Eskimos*, D. Freuchen, Editor. *The World Publishing Company, Cleveland, Ohio, 1961*). Fortunately the foods containing carbohydrate are economical. In every underdeveloped nation, where large numbers of people subsist on very limited amounts of money, the percentage of calories in the diet derived from carbohydrates rises.

As natural or political crises occur and famine ensues, the percentage of carbohydrates in the diet usually rises still further as total caloric intake per capita decreases. Eventually, of course, a point is reached where starvation supervenes. The reverse is true when nations become more affluent. Under these conditions people progressively increase the percentage of fat and protein calories, as well as the total number of calories in their diet.

J. Yudkin (*Lancet 1, 645 (1956)*; *2, 155 (1957)*; *2, 4 (1964)*) has called attention to the increased use of sugar in the diet of nations as they become more affluent. This increase in sweet foods generally is supplied by highly purified items which have lost most or all of their accompanying nutrients. Furthermore, as the consumption of sweets increases, the use of complex carbohydrates (starches) declines proportionately, so the result is a marked decrease in the ratio of complex to simple sugars. This change in the *source* of carbohydrate had been associated statistically with a higher incidence of atherosclerosis and experimentally with a change in blood lipids (Yudkin and J. Roddy, *Lancet 2, 6 (1964)*; M. A. Antar, M. A. Ohlson, and R. E. Hodges, *Am. J. Clin. Nutrition 14, 169 (1964)*; A. M. Cohen, *Am. Heart J.* **65,** *291* (*1963*)). It has been reported that an increase in the portion of carbohydrates supplied as sucrose is followed by a marked rise in serum triglyceride concentration and by a lesser increase in cholesterol concentration. Substitution of starch for sugar has the opposite effect (P. T. Kuo and D. R. Bassett, *Ann. Int. Med.* **62,** *1199* (*1965*); M. Winitz, J. Graff, and D. A. Seedman, *Arch. Biochem. Biophys.* **108,** *576* (*1964*)).

Carbohydrates also have a number of physiologic functions. Their antiketogenic effect is well known, but the quantity required for this purpose is small (J. L. Gamble, G. S. Ross, and F. F. Tisdall, *J. Biol. Chem.* **57,** *633* (*1923*). Similarly, carbohydrates have the ability to conserve water and electrolytes even when supplied in amounts approximating only 100 g. per day (W. L. Bloom and G. J. Azar, *Arch. Int. Med.* **112,** *333* (*1963*). The protein sparing effect of carbohydrates has been recognized in animal husbandry for many years. For man, this is particularly important in situations where food supplies are scarce, not only in planning for people of underdeveloped nations but also for such emergency situations as survival rations, problems of space craft feeding, and military missions. The Food and Nutrition Board (*Recommended Dietary Allowances, Sixth Revised Edition. National Academy of Sciences-National Research Council, Washington, D.C. 1964*) suggests that a normal adult requires approximately 500 carbohydrate calories daily.

At the present time there is a flurry of interest in a popularized diet scheme which is intended for correction of obesity (*The Drinking Man's Diet, vide infra*). Most of the publicity surrounding this dietary approach does not have the sanction of the medical profession, although there are some scientists and practitioners who endorse this method. Diets of this type all are based on the *principle of carbohydrate restriction*.

We know this diet was tried more than 100 years ago (and perhaps long before that). Its reappearance now is in remarkably similar form.

An ear, nose, and throat specialist named William Harvey, of London, chanced to attend a lecture in Paris given by the famous Claude Bernard. Mention was made of the role of the liver in secreting glucose. Harvey, who was already aware of the effect of an "animal diet" in reducing the polyuria of patients with diabetes, was struck by the similarity between common obesity and the obesity which accompanied certain forms of diabetes mellitus. Apparently it was this which prompted him to prescribe for one of his very obese (and deaf) patients a diet furnishing "at least 24 oz. of meat, fish and poultry" and permitting some alcoholic beverages but restricting sweets and farinaceous foods. The patient, a Mr. William Banting, not only lost weight but regained his hearing. He became so impressed that he published and popularized this diet in 1863. Thus the low carbohydrate diet was introduced to the public in a manner not totally unlike the recent introduction of "The Drinking Man's Diet" (J. Alsop, *McCalls*, **138,** *May* (*1965*); R. Wernick, *Saturday Evening Post* **84,** (*1965*)).

From time to time claims are made, usually by lay persons, which cannot be totally supported by fact. These include the idea that "calories don't count" or that a person can "Eat, Eat, Eat Your Pounds Away," (G. Trotta, *Harper's Bazaar* **72,** *July* (*1965*)). A number of serious scientists have pondered the apparent loss of weight which *initially* follows the use of a low carbohydrate diet. Indeed A. W. Pennington (*Am. J. Clin. Nutrition* **1,** *100* (*1953*)) was so firmly convinced that obesity resulted not from excessive calories but from eating the wrong foods, *e.g.* carbohydrates, that he published many articles on the subject. Also, A. Kekwick and G. L. S. Pawan (*Metabolism* **6,** *447* (*1957*)) studied obese subjects who were fed a constant caloric intake but with varying sources of nutrients, largely carbohydrate or protein or fat. They reported that subjects given the high fat diet lost weight most rapidly and that those given the high carbohydrate diet lost weight least rapidly. Unfortunately their studies were of relatively short duration (ten to 21 days).

Other investigators who fed similar diets for longer periods of time have shown that weight loss, in the final analysis, is a result of caloric deficit (T. R. E. Pilkington, H. Gainsborough, V. M. Rosenoer, and M. Carey, *Lancet* **1**, *856* (*1960*); E. S. Olesen and F. Quaade, *Ibid*. **1**, *1048* (*1960*)). It is true that temporary shifts in weight did occur in these studies when fat or carbohydrate predominated in the diet. In almost every instance carbohydrates resulted in a slower rate of loss or even a slight gain of weight for a few days, whereas fats resulted in a more rapid loss of weight for a few days. Generally these departures from the general slope of weight loss were of modest degree and of brief duration. The final conclusion was that weight loss occurs as a result of accumulated caloric deficit. Yudkin (*Ibid*. **2**, *939* (*1960*)) observed that six persons fed a low carbohydrate diet lost weight *because they ate fewer calories* than before.

Although a few scientists have suggested that carbohydrate is nonessential in the human diet (G. M. Briggs, in *Nutrition Reviews* **23**, *95* (*1965*); O. Mickelsen, *Nutrition Science and You. National Science Teachers Association, Washington, D.C., 1964*) the metabolic consequences of complete abstinence from carbohydrate are seemingly undesirable. A number of scientists have referred to the Eskimos as an example of people who, formerly, habitually and voluntarily ate almost no carbohydrate. Actually, when one considers their manner of processing food, it seems possible that their carbohydrate intake was a little higher than we had previously surmised. Fresh frozen meat contains considerably more

glycogen than that which has been allowed to remain at body temperature for some time. Since much of the Eskimos' hunting was done in sub-zero weather, and since they usually butchered their animals on the spot, quick freezing was the inevitable result. Furthermore, the Eskimos customarily ate a considerable portion of their meat in the raw frozen state, and hence may have derived more glycogen from it than we who purchase our meat through commercial sources.

Another curious custom of the Eskimos could have increased the amount of carbohydrate in their animal foods. They prepared a certain number of "delicacies" by permitting a whole seal carcass or whole bird carcasses, encased in a seal skin along with a thick layer of blubber, to "ferment" during the short summer season and then to freeze solid during the winter. These foods then were eaten raw, viscera and all, with great enjoyment. Freuchen (*loc. cit.*) describes the various portions of these fermented birds and seals as having unusual and delightful flavors and colors. For example, one portion might be green and taste like cheddar cheese, and another might be "very sweet" and of strong flavor.

Of course it is impossible to know whether the growth of bacteria and yeasts did convert some amino acids into carbohydrates, but this seems a possibility. Alternatively, the sweetness could come from free glycerol. A final point with regard to the Eskimos seems particularly pertinent. They considered obesity to be a sign of great beauty, and hence it was both fashionable and common to be obese. If, as some authorities would have us believe, the Eskimos ate a strictly protein and fat diet, and if this type of diet will not support obesity, then some other explanation must be sought.

Complete lack of carbohydrate in the diet has been tolerated by healthy people for rather long periods of time. W. S. McClellan and E. F. DuBois (*J. Biol. Chem.* **87**, *651* (*1930*)) and E. Tolstoi (*Ibid*. **83**,

753 (1929)) described two subjects who ate nothing but meat and fat for a period of an entire year. Both these subjects were scientists who had lived in the Arctic, hence they accepted this form of diet without great distaste. There were some minor periods of distress, including irregularities of intestinal function, but the men were able to pursue their usual activities with little difficulty.

It was found, however, that they had a minor increase in the concentration of non-protein nitrogen and a transient rise in uric acid nitrogen in their blood, and some acetone in their urine. It was also noted that their serum "showed a visible lipemia." Measurements of cholesterol indicated that values rose as high as 800 mg. per 100 ml. in one subject and 315 mg. per 100 ml. in the other, with a downward trend as time passed. The lipemia suggests that their triglycerides were high, but measurements for this were not readily available at that time. There are certain similarities between diets without carbohydrate and starvation. Bloom and Azar (*loc. cit.*) have observed that "carbohydrate deficiency" results in loss of water and electrolytes, ketosis, and subjective symptoms of fatigue. Apparently the two subjects in McClellan's study did not experience fatigue and one must assume that the Eskimos of the past were not affected by fatigue.

Obviously man *can* survive for long periods of time without carbohydrates, but this source of food does prevent ketosis, it conserves electrolytes, it spares protein, and it decreases the need for the high fat diet which would otherwise be necessary to provide adequate calories. Furthermore, carbohydrates, which are generally considered to be very pleasant, are not in themselves "fattening." In view of the relationship between hyperlipidemia and hyperuricemia on one hand as accompaniments of a low carbohydrate diet, and potential increase in the atherosclerotic process on the other hand, it would seem wise to retain the time-honored practice of including not only protein and fat but also carbohydrate in the diet. This should include not only normal diets but also those designed for weight reduction (*Diseases of Metabolism, G. G. Duncan, Editor. W. B. Saunders Co., Philadelphia, 1964*). Attempts by journalists and other persons unskilled in scientific methods to treat the general public could result in considerably more harm than good.

CHAPTER IV

PRESENT KNOWLEDGE OF FAT

JAMES F. MEAD, PH.D.

Fat is an important human dietary component (1) by virtue of its high fuel value, (2) because of the palatability that fat imparts to food, (3) because of the "essential" fatty acids in natural fats, and (4) because fats are carriers of the fat soluble vitamins. Fat is the most important form of energy storage in the animal body because of its quantity, high caloric value (more than twice that of carbohydrate), and convenient storage with minimum weight and without appreciable amounts of water or minerals.

The optimal amount of fat in the diet cannot be stated with exactness; certainly wide variations are compatible with health. The National Research Council in its 1948 *Recommended Daily Dietary Allowances* recommended that the average diet should contain 20 to 25 per cent of its calories as fat, and that for active persons with a 4,500 calorie intake and for children and adolescents, 30 to 35 per cent of the caloric intake could be in the form of fat (*Nutrition Reviews* **6**, *319* (*1948*)). These figures are supported by the British Medical Association Committee on Nutrition (*Ibid.* **6**, *191* (*1948*)) and are compatible with the recommendations of the American Medical Association's Council on Foods and Nutrition (*Ibid.* **21**, *36* (*1963*)). Of the approximately 100 g. of fat recommended by these diets, some one-third to one-half would normally be in the form of "visible fats," such as butter, margarine, and other shortenings.

The possibility that a further reduction in dietary fat might be beneficial was raised by the epidemiological studies of A. Keys and his collaborators, carried out over several years, and indicating that populations subsisting on diets with 8 to 14 per cent of the calories supplied as fat had average serum cholesterol values 25 to 50 per cent lower than those from countries in which fat accounted for 38 to 41 per cent of the calories (*Nutrition Reviews* **14**, *67* (*1956*)). However, such discussions of the exact amount of fat in the diet of the general public become less meaningful in the light of the results of M. J. Albrink and others, which show that a decrease in dietary fat is accompanied by an increase in carbohydrate which may correlate with a rise in blood triglycerides, a factor which may correlate with coronary heart disease as well as does serum cholesterol (*Ibid.* **20**, *233* (*1962*)). Since both total serum cholesterol and serum triglycerides actually reflect concentrations of the lipoproteins that appear to be related in some as yet unknown manner to the incidence of atherosclerotic heart disease (*Ibid.* **21**, *36* (*1963*)), it would appear that in the matter of dietary fat, as in many other affairs, extremes of both sorts should be avoided, particularly since rigorous exclusion of fat from the diet may result in the loss of accompanying lipid-soluble micronutrients, including the "essential fatty acids."

More to the point, evidence has accumulated for several years that the type of fat consumed may be of importance. On a diet containing 20 per cent fat, rats had the best growth rates when saturated fatty acids accounted for 30 per cent of the diet (*Nutrition Reviews* **14**, *221* (*1956*)). That growth rate may not be an entirely reliable criterion, however, is indicated by the experiments of H. J. Thomasson (*J. Nutrition* **57**, *17* (*1955*)), who found that, in rats fed high fat diets, greater longevity was associated with lower growth rates. In many studies carried out with human subjects and experimental animals, investigators have found that higher proportions of polyunsaturated fatty acids in the dietary fat are associated with lower serum cholesterol (*Nutrition Reviews* **15,** *1* (*1957*)). This cholesterol-lowering effect takes place even with a relatively high dietary fat content, and is brought about by such fats as fish oils and seed oils as well as the more highly purified polyunsaturated fatty acids used in experimental procedures (*Ibid.* **14,** *327* (*1956*); **18,** *9* (*1960*); **19,** *117* (*1961*)). In a more quantitative light, it has been suggested that a 15 per cent reduction in serum cholesterol can be achieved by an increase in the ratio of dietary polyunsaturated to saturated fatty acids from the usual 0.4 to 1.1 or more (N. Jolliffe *et al., N. Y. State J. Med.* **63,** *69* (*1963*)). The mechanism or mechanisms by which such effects are achieved, however, are still not at all certain.

Fat Absorption. In normal individuals, fat is absorbed to an extent of 95 per cent or better except for fully saturated glycerides, which are rather poorly absorbed (*Nutrition Reviews* **3,** *278* (*1945*); **5,** *155* (*1947*); **14,** *200* (*1956*)). In severe malnutrition (*Ibid.* **15,** *36* (*1957*)), obstructive jaundice (*Ibid.* **15,** *167* (*1957*)), and certain other diseases, fat absorption is poor and steatorrhea results (less than 90 per cent absorption). This condition may sometimes be alleviated by feeding emulsifying agents such as Tween 80 (polyoxyethylene sorbitan monooleate) (*Ibid.* **7,** *205* (*1949*)).

Present theories of fat absorption have been reviewed by J. R. Senior (*J. Lipid Res.* **5,** *495* (*1964*)), K. J. Isselbacher (*Fed. Proc.* **24,** *16* (*1965*)), and others. Fat is largely hydrolyzed to fatty acids and monoglycerides by pancreatic lipase in the small intestine, where emulsification takes place with the aid of bile salts, ultimately producing micelles, which are absorbed through the brush border of the intestinal mucosa. During passage through the intestinal epithelial cells, triglycerides are resynthesized from the fatty acids and monoglycerides with utilization of some additional glycerol derived largely from carbohydrate. The triglycerides thus formed appear in the lymph as high molecular weight, low density lipoproteins, or chylomicrons, which are transported to the blood via the thoracic duct.

Other fat soluble substances are also absorbed with the triglycerides and, indeed, triglyceride absorption is necessary for efficient absorption of these substances. The extent of absorption of cholesterol varies widely depending on the species of animal and the accompanying diet. In the presence of oleic acid, it may be absorbed to an extent of 50 per cent but when fed alone its absorption is much poorer. Cholesterol esters are completely hydrolyzed in the small intestine but appear in the lymph about 70 per cent esterified and are transported in chylomicrons to the liver where the cholesterol is largely converted to bile acids. The bile acids are then reexcreted into the small intestine and reabsorbed with the products of fat digestion in a cyclic process. This enterohepatic cycle of bile acids and cholesterol provides a means of regulation of cholesterol synthesis in the liver, which is under negative feedback control. It is in part for this reason that elimination of cholesterol from the diet is not entirely effective in regulation of blood cholesterol (*Nutrition Reviews* **16,** *42* (*1958*)).

Metabolism. As a result of intensive research efforts by many laboratories, the mechanisms of biosynthesis and oxidation of the fatty acids and other lipids are fairly well understood, and some knowledge of the regulatory mechanisms of these processes has become available.

Lipids appearing in the blood from the lymph are transported, mainly as chylomicrons, to the tissues, largely the liver and adipose tissue, for metabolism and storage. In the liver mitochondria, the fatty acids are activated as thioesters of coenzyme A, a derivative of pantothenic acid. In this activated form they can be used for synthesis of various complex lipids, or oxidized for energy production. In the beta-oxidation scheme as elucidated in the laboratories of F. Lynen (*Ann. Rev. Biochem.* **24,** *653* (*1955*)) and D. E. Green (in *Lipid Metabolism, K. Bloch, Editor. John Wiley & Sons, Inc., New York, 1960*) and others, the acyl CoA derivatives are oxidized to acetyl CoA with production of energy in the form of ATP. The acetyl CoA can then be oxidized to carbon dioxide and water via the Krebs cycle with production of considerably more ATP, or it can be condensed to acetoacetate. Particularly in diabetes and starvation, acetoacetate, or other "ketone bodies," increase greatly in concentration, in large part because of the greatly increased metabolism of fat in these conditions. It is of interest that acetoacetate is also the starting point for biosynthesis of cholesterol, which is related to a high fat diet.

The deposition of fat in adipose tissue is in part under control of dietary (and hence blood) fat and of dietary carbohydrate, while its release from adipose tissue (as the fatty acid-albumin complex) is under control of various hormones, particularly epinephrine, and of carbohydrate (*Nutrition Reviews* **20,** *154* (*1962*)). Thus, with high dietary carbohydrate, in the normal individual, mobilization from adipose tissue is inhibited, probably as a result of esterification of fatty acids with α-glyceryl phosphate formed from the carbohydrate in the adipose tissue, and, consequently, fatty acid oxidation is decreased. With fasting, a high fat diet, or in diabetes, this type of control is lost and there is increased mobilization and consequent oxidation of fatty acids.

The mechanism of biosynthesis of fatty acids has recently been elucidated in the laboratories of S. J. Wakil, Lynen, and others (*Nutrition Reviews* **21,** *155* (*1963*)) and involves, as a first step, the carboxylation of acetyl coenzyme A to malonyl coenzyme A, the fundamental building unit, in a reaction involving biotin as a coenzyme (*Nutrition Reviews* **17,** *59* (*1959*); **20,** *143* (*1962*)). Repeated condensation of these units attached to a protein carrier results in the formation of long chain fatty acids. Fatty acid biosynthesis is also under control of several factors, including dietary. It is increased with dietary carbohydrate, which provides citrate, a direct stimulator of acetyl CoA carboxylase and source of extramitochrondrial acetyl CoA, extramitochondrial reductive power as TNPH (particularly from the malic enzyme), and alpha-glyceryl phosphate for the formation of glycerides from the fatty acids (*Ibid.* **21,** *247* (*1963*); **22,** *268* (*1964*)). Fasting, diabetes, and high fat diets decrease fatty acid biosynthesis, in part because of the direct inhibition of acetyl CoA carboxylase by long chain acyl CoA.

The acyl CoA thus formed may be incorporated into phospholipids or triglycerides, particularly during periods of high energy intake, and stored in adipose tissue.

Thus it is becoming apparent that energy metabolism, involving mainly carbohydrate and fat, is carried on in a complex series of interrelated reactions under control of many factors, particularly dietary, but including hormonal and nervous. As our knowledge of the reactions and their regulation increases we should be in an increasingly better position to understand the normal processes and the diseases in which they are involved.

Chapter V

REDUCTION OF NITROGEN DEFICITS IN SURGICAL PATIENTS MAINTAINED BY INTRAVENOUS ALIMENTATION

Stanley Levey, Ph.D.

There are numerous patients who take nothing by mouth because of an inability to ingest or retain food or because their physicians withhold all oral feedings to allow the digestive tract to remain at rest. While their intake of nutrients has been reduced to zero, the daily requirements of these substances proceed at a normal or even accelerated pace. The patient still needs water, electrolytes, calories, and nitrogen. Otherwise, increasing deficits develop. Intravenously administered electrolytes and glucose solutions are commonly used to reduce the deficits of water and electrolytes. To prevent accumulation of large nitrogen deficits in the non-ingesting patient it is necessary to provide all the components required for the formation of tissue. These include adequate amounts of calories, electrolytes, water, and all the necessary amino acids and vitamins.

Hydrolyzates of nutritionally good proteins provide a good source of utilizable nitrogen for the non-ingesting patient. When such preparations are made up in 10 per cent hexose solutions, they yield about 550 calories per liter, including the nitrogen calories. Two liters of such solutions supply the equivalent of 75 g. of protein and about 1,100 calories per day. Increasing the caloric intake by administering more of the fluids increases the danger of overloading the body with fluid. The development of fat emulsions that can be given intravenously allows administration of larger caloric intakes without giving excessive fluid. Such emulsions yield about 1.5 calories per milliliter.

Over a period of years, W. E. Abbott and associates (W. D. Holden, H. Krieger, S. Levey, and Abbott, *Ann. Surg.* **146,** *563* (*1957*); Abbott, Levey, and Krieger, *Metab-*olism **8,** *847* (*1959*); Abbott and K. Albertsen, *Nutritio et Dieta* **5,** *339* (*1963*)) have carried out studies which indicate that the nitrogen deficit that occurs following uncomplicated surgical procedures is mainly the result of a decreased intake of nitrogen and calories, and by adequate nutritional maintenance of patients during the immediate postoperative period, these deficits can be minimized or, in some cases, eliminated.

The magnitude of the nitrogen deficit that occurs in patients maintained on poor nutritional intakes following surgical procedures is related to the severity of the surgical procedure. In general, it is greater following serious surgical operations and less following minor surgery. For this reason, Krieger, Abbott, Levey, and Holden (*Gastroenterology* **33,** *807* (*1957*)) studied the effects of levels of intravenous alimentation on a series of male patients, each undergoing a major surgical operation: a subtotal gastric resection. The patients were maintained on the various regimens on the day of operation plus the next four postoperative days, and the nitrogen balance was calculated for the period. Group One consisted of ten patients who were given, intravenously, solutions containing 10 per cent carbohydrate and electrolytes. For a 70 kg. man this is about 900 calories per day. With such a nutritional intake the average deficit for the five day period was 57.9 g., or an average daily deficit of 11.6 g.

Group Two consisted of ten patients who received a modest intake of calories (average 23 kilocalories per kg. per day) and nitrogen (average 0.17 g. per kg. per day). The intravenous alimentation consisted of amino acid solutions and hexose, with the necessary electrolytes added to the various solutions.

The average five day nitrogen deficit for this group of patients was 38.2 g., or an average daily nitrogen deficit of 7.6 g. per day. Thus, giving the patient nitrogen and a modest caloric intake (1,610 calories per 70 kg. man) reduced the nitrogen deficit about one-third of that on the nitrogen free intake.

The third group consisted of ten patients who received a good caloric and nitrogen intake (38 calories and 0.28 g. of nitrogen per kilogram per day). The increased caloric intake was achieved by using a fat emulsion in addition to hexose and protein hydrolyzate. For a 70 kg. man this would be 19.6 g. of nitrogen and 2,450 calories. The five day nitrogen deficit for this group was 7.3 g., or an average daily deficit of 1.5 g.

This series of studies indicates that administration of an adequate caloric intake plus nitrogen to a patient following major surgery minimizes the nitrogen deficit. Also, the loss of body weight for the latter group of patients was small, about one pound during the five day period compared with values of seven to nine pounds for patients who were receiving only hexose and electrolytes.

Recently, L. B. Wadstrom and P. E. Wirklund (*Acta Chir. Scandinav., Suppl.* **325,** *50 (1964)*) also reported on the effect of caloric supplementation on the nitrogen balance of patients following an uncomplicated cholecystectomy. The patients were maintained on intravenous feeding during the 48 hour period of study, which started at 8 a.m. on the day of operation. Three groups of female patients were studied. Group One contained ten patients who received 10 calories per kilogram per day in the form of carbohydrate solutions and no nitrogen. The average two day postoperative deficit for this group was 11.9 g. The second group consisted of nine patients, each receiving 10 calories per kilogram and 0.1 g. of nitrogen. The total caloric intake included the sum of carbohydrate and nitrogen calories. These patients showed an average 48 hour nitrogen deficit of 4.8 g.

The third group consisted of nine patients who received 35 calories per kilogram and 0.1 g. of nitrogen. The average caloric intake for this group was 2,200 calories per day, with the calories being derived from carbohydrate, amino acids, and a fat emulsion. The fat was given at a level of 1 g. per kg. The average 48 hour nitrogen deficit for the patients in Group Three was 1.2 g., or 0.6 g. per day, indicating that they were approaching balance in spite of the operative procedure. Two of the nine patients showed positive nitrogen balances during the period.

Both series of studies indicate that the nitrogen deficit which occurs in the uncomplicated patient following surgical operations may be largely due to poor nutritional intake during this period. Patients who receive only carbohydrate solutions with or without supplementary electrolytes must develop nitrogen deficits, since their intake of protein or amino acids is zero. Those who receive protein hydrolyzates along with carbohydrate have decreased nitrogen deficits, but usually they do not receive sufficient calories to reduce the nitrogen deficit to a minimum. While it is possible to give adequate amounts of nitrogen by vein without overloading the patient with fluid, the provision of sufficient calories is much more difficult. Now that fat emulsions which can be given by vein are available, it is possible to provide complete nutritional intakes, including vitamins, nitrogen, calories, electrolytes, and trace elements parenterally.

While it is possible to minimize or even negate, in some cases, the nitrogen deficit which may occur in postoperative patients along with the loss in body weight, it is difficult to demonstrate that this is beneficial in the non-debilitated patient. However, P. R. Cannon (*Some Pathologic Consequences of Protein and Amino Acid Deficiencies. Charles C Thomas, Springfield, Illinois, 1948*) has documented the increased incidence of complications which occur in patients who have a protein deficiency. These studies would suggest that proper parenteral alimentation in the postoperative patient is a valuable adjunct to successful surgery.

Chapter VI

PRESENT KNOWLEDGE OF INTRAVENOUS FAT EMULSIONS

Richard J. Jones, M.D.

It has been widely appreciated for many years that intravenous or parenteral alimentation could never be complete without including fat in the infusion. Without the high caloric value of fat it is virtually impossible to get enough calories into the patient to permit a positive nitrogen balance. Because emulsified fat exerts no osmotic effect, its concentration can be increased to 15 to 20 per cent of the infusion without running into the chemical thrombophlebitis induced by concentrated solutes.

Homologous chyle from healthy subjects would offer one approach to such a therapy, but this is hardly practical. Lipemic plasma or mother's milk have been used intravenously without serious side effects, but the caloric content of such material is far less than can be achieved by artificial fat emulsions. However, with the vegetable oil emulsions that had been prepared acute toxic effects remained too frequent to encourage their use until about nine years ago (*Nutrition Reviews* **16**, *164* (*1958*). An excellent review by R. P. Geyer (*Physiol. Rev.* **40**, *150* (*1960*), a colloquium on intravenous feeding held in London in 1962 (*Nutritio et Dieta* **5**, *295* (*1963*)), and a symposium on intravenous fat emulsions in a recent issue of *Am. J. Clin. Nutrition* (*16, 1* (*1965*)) are recommended for complete coverage of this subject.

The ideal fat emulsion for intravenous use should resemble natural chyle closely in containing lipid particles a very few microns in diameter, which are in stable suspension, sterile, and capable of complete metabolic utilization. It should maintain all these characteristics for a substantial period of time so that shipping and storing will not spoil it for use. Finally, of course, it must not be toxic. Most emulsions can now be made with proper emulsifiers to have fat particles less than 1 μ. in diameter in a stable, sterile emulsion.

The search for nontoxic phospholipid and other emulsifiers has been fairly well completed, and appropriate conditions of preparation and storage are now well established. The high incidence of acute toxic reactions has been drastically reduced: although they have not been excluded or even reduced to a negligible figure, such side effects as continue to occur are not severe. The chief deterrent to the widespread use of this form of nourishment for prolonged periods is the side effects which develop after a series of five or more daily infusions which may relate in part to the accumulation in certain cells of an indigestible pigment.

Short chain triglycerides, such as tributyrin and trinorvalerin, induce acute changes in pulse rate, blood pressure, and respiration. Trivalerin has a negative inotropic effect on the heart and induces vasodilatation. The longer chain triglycerides, however, avoid these difficulties to a considerable extent, provided a proper emulsifying agent is used. An important advance in the preparation of benign emulsions was the demonstration that soybean phosphatides, used as emulsifying agents, were only capable of inducing blood pressure changes when they had been oxidized by exposure to air (Geyer, D. M. Watkin, L. W. Matthews, and F. J. Stare, *J. Lab. Clin. Med.* **34**, *688* (*1949*)).

Further experience with these emulsifying agents has only emphasized the importance of careful fractionation of soybean phosphatides for removal of pharmacologically active fractions, if acute toxic effects are to be minimized. Egg phosphatides seem to require less purification (O. Schuberth and K. A. Wretlind, *Acta Chir. Scandinav. Suppl.* **278,** *1* (*1961*)). "Colloidal reactions," characterized by back or chest pain with dyspnea and cyanosis, once common with early preparations, have been all but eliminated, presumably by the more highly purified fats used in the emulsion today.

Acute effects which are still seen include fever, usually low grade, flushing of the skin, and, rarely, hypotension. The reason for the fever remains fairly obscure. It has been argued that it is not due to the bacterial or chemical pyrogens that plagued many early efforts at other forms of intravenous therapy, and yet it has become less severe, although still the most frequent side effect, with the latest preparations containing the purest ingredients.

The remaining circulatory effects are largely attributed to changes in the microcirculation: alterations in the shape of erythrocytes, adherence of granulocytes to capillary endothelium, and transient slowing of the capillary flow have been observed in the rabbit ear chamber (P. I. Bronemark and J. Lindström, *Circulation Res.* **15,** *124* (*1964*)). These investigators were not impressed with any unusual aggregation of erythrocytes or "sludging" of the blood which had been noted earlier by A. V. Williams, A. C. Higgenbotham, and M. H. Knisely (*Angiology* **8,** *29* (*1957*)). In any case, a diminished oxygen tension in the myocardium and peripheral tissues has been demonstrated during hyperlipemia by several workers (C. R. Joyner, O. Horwitz, and P. G. Williams, *Circulation* **22,** *901* (*1960*); T. J. Regan *et al.*, *Ibid.* **23,** *55* (*1961*)).

Undesirable late effects, seen after repeated infusions, are more frequent, less well understood, and therefore a greater bar to widespread use of these agents. These effects, however, depend to a large extent upon the dose and type of fat emulsion employed. Although many other combinations have been studied, there are essentially two

fat emulsions which have reached the stage of commercial availability: a 15 per cent cottonseed oil emulsion employing 1.2 per cent soybean lecithin and 0.3 per cent polyoxyethyleneoxypropylene as emulsifying agents, available in the U.S., and a 20 per cent soybean oil emulsion, employing as emulsifiers egg lecithin and glycerol, made in Sweden. The analysis of trace materials in these and many new combinations may permit further understanding of some of the more lasting effects of lipid infusions (A. Rose, N. Pelick, F. M. Angeloni, and M. E. Miller, *Am. J. Clin. Nutrition* **16,** *4* (*1965*)).

These effects, which become apparent after several daily infusions of about 2.0 g. fat per kilogram per day, include the development of a normochromic, normocytic (probably hemolytic) anemia, leucocytosis, hemorrhagic diathesis, alterations in the serum protein pattern, disturbances in liver function—occasionally to the point of jaundice, peptic ulceration of the stomach and duodenum, and other less specific gastrointestinal complaints. The "overloading syndrome" is characterized by fever, headache, hyperirritability, and any or all of the preceding symptoms, often with a persisting hyperlipemia. These late symptoms are reported to be much less frequent and less severe with the soybean oil than with the cottonseed oil emulsion.

In comparing these two with newer experimental emulsions given as large daily infusions to groups of dogs, A. R. Vela *et al.* (*Am. J. Clin. Nutrition* **16,** *80* (*1965*)) showed that a 15 per cent cottonseed oil emulsion with polyethylene glycol monoglyceride and other purified emulsifiers could be given to dogs for six weeks without apparent ill effects. In human beings, however, several acute but mild reactions occurred in six to eight carcinomatous patients tested. It was concluded that no truly innocuous emulsion had yet been developed.

Of more interest is the apparently inevitable involvement of the liver and the reticuloendothelial system in all animals receiving repeated intravenous infusions of fat emulsion. Microscopic study of the organs of such animals reveals the appearance of an "intravenous fat pigment" in Küpffer cells, hepatic cells, and reticuloendothelial cells of the spleen (C. E. Meyer, J. A. Fancher, P. E. Schurr, and H. D. Webster, *Metabolism* **6**, *591* (*1957*)). This intracytoplasmic material is sudanophilic, anisotropic, fluorescent, iron-negative and, therefore, seems to be a lipoid-pigment complex of some kind.

This complex is frequently associated with multiple microscopic lipoid fibrogranulomata which develop in the liver and spleen of these animals. It is not always evident by light microscopy after administration of the soybean oil emulsion, but can be observed with the electron microscope in all treated animals. It appears with much lower frequency and intensity following infusion of the soybean oil emulsion than after the cottionseed oil or similar emulsions. Its amount varies with the dose as well as the type of material infused, but has little relationship to the acute toxic manifestations, the type of emulsifier used, or the fat particle size. It does not appear after emulsions are administered orally, so it must be caused by some trace material which is not absorbed from the gastrointestinal tract (perhaps gossypol, a lipid soluble hepatotoxic phenolic pigment in cottonseed), or the formation of some protein-lipid aggregate or, more likely, an oxidized lipid complex which is ingested but poorly handled by these cells. The pigment complex does not disappear with time, but the pigment granules become larger, persisting for at least 18 months and probably for the lifetime of the animal (S. W. Thompson *et al.*, *Am. J. Clin. Nutrition* **16**, *43* (*1965*)).

Even after the soybean oil emulsions are administered, ultrastructural changes in the cellular organelles are regularly seen (H. Sasaki, F. Schaffner, Thompson, and R. D. Hunt, *Ibid.* **16**, *37* (*1965*)). The pigment granules, though small, are associated with sites of alkaline phosphatase activity in the cell, and after a month's time can be seen to have increased in size and to be surrounded sometimes by a single membrane. In addition, a distortion and dilatation of the rough endoplasmic reticulum occurs, with partial loss of ribosomes and hypertrophy of the Golgi apparatus.

Although these findings closely resemble the abnormalities seen in the fine structure of the liver in choline deficiency, choline supplementation does not seem to prevent their development. While the changes do not appear to reflect serious damage to liver function, and may not be considered as sufficient reason for rejecting all use of intravenous fat emulsions, their innocence cannot be assumed, since they do persist for the duration of the test animal's life.

Although it has not been definitely related to the symptoms or pathologic findings mentioned above, a plasma element found in some patients has been reported to break the emulsion and allow the formation of insoluble calcium soaps *in vitro*. H. LeVeen, P. Giordano, and A. Johnson (*Am. J. Clin. Nutrition* **16**, *129* (*1965*)) have studied this phenomenon, which does not occur with normal serum, and present evidence to suggest that it is due to a serum globulin. Eighty-five per cent of patients with an elevated erythrocyte sedimentation rate carried this element in their plasma. So far no successful means has been found to correct this tendency, although it must also be said that any significance it may have to events *in vivo* remains to be established.

As far as disposition of the intravascular fat is concerned, studies on its disappearance from the blood of patients suggest at least two exponential components, one of which is so rapid as to suggest reticuloendothelial phagocytosis for a substantial fraction of the material, a slower uptake curve being attributed to the liver. Animal studies have revealed early uptake of labeled fat emulsions by spleen, liver, and lung, over 25 per cent remaining in these organs after an hour. Yet there is extensive evidence for the fact that intravenous artificial fat emulsions are metabolized as well as an orally administered preparation. In fact, studies of the fat particles present at the end of an infusion of the cottonseed oil emulsion, and four hours later, show that these artificial chylomicrons have about the same proportions of protein, cholesterol, and phospholipid as naturally occurring chylomicrons seen after a fat meal.

In conclusion, it must still be said that artificial fat emulsions are not yet perfected to the point where they can be recommended for general use in patients requiring temporary parenteral nutrition. On the other hand, continued improvement over the last 20 years in the purity of the oils and the emulsifiers used has reduced the incidence and intensity of side effects so that there is reason to hope that further understanding may soon lead to their ultimate exclusion. The problem posed by the persistent intracellular changes that appear following infusion of all emulsions so far studied remains a thorny one. Since there does seem to be a difference between preparations in this manifestation, there is room even here for optimism.

CHAPTER VII

PRESENT KNOWLEDGE OF SPECIFIC DYNAMIC ACTION

WENDELL H. GRIFFITH, PH.D. AND
HELEN M. DYER, PH.D.

Specific dynamic action (SDA) was discussed briefly in relation to "the present knowledge of calories in human nutrition" (*Nutrition Reviews* **4,** *34 (1946)*). In the next year original data and critical discussions of the literature on the mechanisms of SDA, with special reference to the effects of vitamins, enzymes, and hormones, appeared (*Research Bulletin 404–418, February 1947– May 1948, University of Missouri, College of Agriculture, Columbia, Missouri*). H. H. Mitchell (*Comparative Nutrition of Man and Domestic Animals, Vol. II. Academic Press, New York, 1962*) devoted two sections to the discussion of past and present knowledge relative to factors affecting the net availability of metabolizable energy and the causation of the SDA of foods.

The classic concept of SDA of foodstuffs (M. Rubner, *Die Gesetze des Energiever- brauchs bei der Ernahrung. Leipzig, 1902*) is apparently true qualitatively, and also quantitatively when each type of foodstuff is administered singly to a fasted subject in the resting state. The extent of the SDA is dependent on 1) the amount of nutrient eaten, 2) the basal metabolism of the subject, and 3) the nutritional state of the subject. If the foodstuff is administered separately as protein, carbohydrate, or fat in a resting subject on a maintenance diet or on a diet with excess calories, then the quantitative values of the SDA change. With a mixed diet of foodstuffs fed to rats the SDA is quantitatively much less than the sum of the SDAs of the component foodstuffs (E. B. Forbes and R. W. Swift, *J. Nutrition* **27,** *453 (1944)*). The significance of SDA in total heat production is said to

have been greatly overemphasized except in the case of ruminants, where the effect is important. However, the use of ruminants for investigations of SDA has been objected to for many reasons, including the presence of parasites in the food and the differences between the amount of food ingested and the amount utilized.

Relatively little is known of the SDA of mixed diets in human nutrition. Determinations of SDA have been confined to adults and are concerned usually with the extra calories produced over the basal expenditure. Relatively few studies involve measurement of the SDA produced by a meal of definite description and few extend over periods of sufficient duration. In man ingesting a mixed diet, high protein was not observed to strain the heat dissipation mechanism of the body (N. Glickman, H. H. Mitchell, E. H. Lambert, and R. W. Keeton, *J. Nutrition* **36,** *41 (1948)*). The quantity of food ingested is more important in heat production than the SDA of the components of the diet, and this effect is related to the previous level of nourishment. After fasting and after starvation the relative SDA of foods is markedly decreased (A. Keys *et al., The Biology of Human Starvation. University of Minnesota Press, Minneapolis, 1950*).

The results of early investigations suggested that the SDA or "wasted" energy comes from so many different reactions of the foodstuffs in the body that they are unmeasurable so far as pinpointing the individual sources of fractions of the energy. Digestion and absorption are included as causing part of the SDA but metabolism of the absorbed products seems to be the greatest source of energy measured as the SDA.

Other aspects of SDA have been considered. J. R. Brobeck's hypothesis (*Proceedings of the Twentieth International Congress of Physiology, p. 133, 1956; Rec. Prog. Hormone Res.* **16**, *439 (1960)*) relating the satiety mechanism with regard to the ingestion of foods to the sensitivity of the hypothalamus has been confirmed (R. Passmore and F. J. Ritchie, *Brit. J. Nutrition* **11**, *79 (1957)*). The mechanism is believed to involve the sensitivity of the hypothalamus to the heat of the SDA of foods. An experiment with goats demonstrated a relationship between the thermoregulatory areas and hypothalamic feeding centers which supported the theory that the SDA of foods acts to evoke cutaneous vasodilation, inhibition of appetite, and induction of satiety (*Nutrition Reviews* **20**, *26 (1962)*). Studies under normal conditions of food intake are indicated with monitoring of temperature changes in preoptic and rostral hypothalmic areas.

In a reinvestigation of one phase of the classical work of Rubner on SDA, the increment in heat production associated with eating a 1,000 Kcal. meal (40 per cent of the calories was protein) and the increment associated with exposure to cold showed summation when human subjects were fed while resting in the cold (E. R. Buskirk, R. H. Thompson, R. Moore, and G. D. Whedon, *Am. J. Clin. Nutrition* **8**, *602 (1960)*). The problem of equivalence of SDA in exercise thermogenesis and cold thermogenesis has been discussed by J. S. Hart (*Transactions of the Sixth Conference on Cold Injury, S. M. Horvath, Editor, p. 271. Josiah Macy, Jr. Foundation, New York, 1960*). The burning of fuel to maintain body temperature during exposure to cold is an essential process that involves muscle work in the form of shivering and, also, a mechanism called "non-shivering thermogenesis." Whether or not any of the

reactions that account for SDA are also used as a source of heat in non-shivering thermogenesis is not known.

SDA has sometimes been regarded as a method of body weight regulation. High protein diets have been recommended for this purpose. In growing rats, total heat production—the difference between caloric intake and the sum of fecal and urinary losses plus body gain—was minimal when the diet contained 25 to 41 per cent of protein and increased at higher and lower dietary protein levels (E. W. Hartsook and T. V. Hershberger, *J. Nutrition* **81**, *209 (1963)*). The data indicated that the trend of total heat production of rats to decrease at a moderate rate with increasing dietary protein is reversed at higher concentration of protein, when the optimal level is clearly exceeded from the standpoint of energy gain. The conclusions were criticized because the assumption had been made that computed differences in heat production among dietary protein groups were more logically ascribable to variation in SDA than to activity of the rats (*Nutrition Reviews* **22**, *156 (1964)*). Two early reports had observed that the SDAs of diets containing varying concentrations of dried extract of whole egg decreased coincidently with every increase in protein until 18 per cent was present, remained constant between 18 and 30 per cent, and increased in diets containing 42 per cent or more of protein (T. S. Hamilton, *J. Nutrition* **17**, *565, 583 (1939)*). At that time the author stated that the higher net energy value of well-balanced diets as compared with diets unbalanced, either because of insufficiency or excess of protein, lies almost entirely in the smaller heat increment of the well-balanced diets.

Weight maintenance was achieved in weanling rats over a wide range of caloric intakes (D. S. Miller and R. R. Payne, *J. Nutrition* **78**, *255 (1962)*). Two young pigs were maintained also at constant weight with diets providing, respectively, 243 and

1,180 Calories per day. The stock diet (low calorie) was mixed with additional carbohydrate to furnish the increased calories so the nitrogen contents were 4.1 and 0.41 per cent respectively. After 40 days the regimens were reversed and body weight was maintained for a similar period. These surprising results could not be accounted for by differences in digestibility, losses in the urine, storage of depot fat, or physical activity. Differences in expired carbon dioxide showed that all the ingested food was being metabolized. It was concluded that food energy may be converted directly into heat. A direct production of heat from fat and carbohydrate would interfere seriously with evaluation of the SDA of proteins in mixed diets indicating that the protein to calorie ratio and caloric intake must be taken into account (Miller and Payne, *Brit. J. Nutrition* **15**, *11 (1961)*).

Reconsideration of observations related to SDA has led to two new concepts to account for this phenomenon: 1) SDA is a result of an imbalance in the diet or of a dietary deficiency, and 2) SDA is the result of wastage of energy of foodstuffs due to the metabolizing of energy-rich compounds to form compounds of lower energy. The second theory involves conversion of metabolites that are in excess of body needs into forms for storage, such as conversion of glucose into glycerol, and into fatty acids in lipogenesis, and synthesis of peptides from amino acids.

Support of the theory that the wasted heat of foodstuffs is due to a deficiency or imbalance in the components of the diet may be found in analysis of most of the experiments in which the SDA of test foodstuffs has been measured.

Relative to the second concept, the free energy of conversion of foodstuffs into storage products must come from the metabolic processes going on in the organism. An approximation of the cost of the conversion of amino acids into proteins indicated that the complete oxidation of a single glucose molecule into carbon dioxide and liquid water yields approximately 700,000 calories of free energy, an amount in the order of magnitude sufficient for the building into proteins of about a hundred amino acid residues (J. A. V. Butler, *Nature* **158**, *153 (1946)*). The specific dynamic action from the standpoint of the second and third laws of thermodynamics has been considered (E. T. Adams, *J. Biol. Chem.* **67**, *XXI–XXII (1926)*). The output of waste heat is increased whenever there is uncoupling of oxidative phosphorylation from oxidation along the electron transport chain. Uncoupling deprives the body of a major source of an energy enrichment process that yields ATP (P. Oesper, in *Phosphorus Metabolism, W. D. McElroy and B. Glass, Editors, Vol. I. p. 523. Johns Hopkins Press, Baltimore, 1951*). Uncoupling agents include normal body constituents, such as thyroxine and calcium. Whether or not uncoupling results in a significant loss of energy as waste heat under ordinary circumstances is not known.

The two newer concepts for explaining the cause of SDA, namely deficient or imbalanced diets, and the waste of energy in the conversion of high energy products of digestion to low energy metabolites deserve further investigation. Of especial interest is an explanation of the failure of many individuals who engage in "luxus consumption" to store additional fat or to gain body weight. Another question that may be worthy of study is whether or not the energy represented by basal metabolism is analogous to that defined as SDA, a form of energy transfer that also is unavailable for doing work.

Chapter VIII

PRESENT KNOWLEDGE OF CEROID PIGMENT

W. Stanley Hartroft, M.D., Ph.D. and E. A. Porta, M.D.

During the past decade or more, reports from a number of laboratories, some dealing with apparently unrelated nutritional conditions, have appeared which have gradually given rise to a number of new fundamental concepts. They are broadly related to the response of a wide variety of tissues to injuries in which nutritional imbalances more often play an important part. The abnormality which these conditions share is the deposition of ceroid pigment. It is an amber material found in unstained sections which cannot be extracted by most commonly employed reagents (*i.e.* alcohol, petroleum ether, acetone, xylol) and which has a strong affinity for lipophilic dyes (Sudan, Oil red O, Sudan Black B, Osmium tetroxide). The pigment is usually classified as a lipochrome and is certainly closely related to, if not identical with, others in this group, such as lipofucsin, hemofucsin, so-called myocardial "wear-tear" or "age" pigment, the pigment found in the muscle in experimental nutritional muscular dystrophy and still other related conditions.

The term ceroid, meaning wax-like (L. cera(wax)) was first introduced almost a quarter century ago (R. D. Lillie *et al., Pub. Health Rep.* **57,** *502* (*1942*)) to describe the alcohol and xylol-insoluble pigment demonstrable in paraffin-imbedded sections of cirrhotic livers of choline deficient rats. It was found in parenchymal cells, in Küpffer cells, and in the fibrous trabeculae. In the latter position it was sometimes contained within macrophages and in other instances was free within collagen bundles. Whatever its position, it stained brilliantly with lipophilic dyes as well as with periodic acid-Schiff reagents (PAS-positive) and a variety of basophilic dyes. The PAS-posi-

tive reaction of ceroid has not infrequently led to the misinterpretation of deposits of pigment as mucopolysaccharide, particularly in studies of atheromata, because ceroid stains are often not prepared. The report of Lillie and co-workers stimulated the interest of other experimental pathologists of nutrition and reawakened morphologic interest in the lipochromes generally.

It is now recognized that the pigment has a wide distribution in both experimental animals and man. In a recent review (W. S. Hartroft and E. A. Porta, *Am. J. Med. Sci.* **250,** *324* (*1965*)), reports were cited in which it has been described not only in livers of rats with a broad spectrum of dietary injuries, but also in uterus, sex glands, spleen, lymph nodes, and adipose tissue of vitamin E deficient rats. It has been found in the adipose tissue of vitamin E deficient chicks and in liver, adrenal glands, and testes of the mouse and in fish liver and spleen under other experimental conditions. It is present in coronary arterial thrombi of rats fed thrombogenic diets and in livers of mice and rats fed the hepatic necrogenic diets of H. P. Himsworth and K. Schwarz (Schwarz, *Proc. Soc. Exp. Biol. Med.* **77,** *818* (*1951*)).

In man, it has been reported in liver, spleen, kidney, adrenal, lymph nodes, esophagus, stomach and small intestine, medium size arteries, venules and capillaries, ovary, uterus, seminal vesicles, skeletal muscle, pituitary, and the central nervous system. It is a relatively early and constant finding in human atheromatous aortas and coronary arteries as well as in occlusive thrombi found obstructing the latter in cases of fatal myocardial infarction. In children, two cases of designated "ceroid-storage disease" have been described with the pigment distributed within liver, spleen, lymph nodes, bone marrow, intestines, and the fat surrounding the thymus. It has been regarded as the end product in some forms of Niemann-Pick disease and has been described in the reticuloendothelial cells in the hemorrhagic diathesis of albinos.

It is prominent in the smooth muscle of the intestinal tract in cystic fibrosis of the pancreas and in biliary atresia, as well as in chronic pancreatitis and certain cases of malabsorption. It is almost constantly found in the human ovary and here can be regarded as a normal occurrence. There are at least a half-dozen reports of its presence in the reticuloendothelial cells of patients given fat emulsions intravenously. We have found it to be regularly demonstrable in most types of cirrhosis, particularly those cases associated with chronic and excessive consumption of alcoholic beverages. From the foregoing it can be seen that the formation of ceroid must represent a fundamental reaction to tissue injury, if on no other grounds than its ubiquity in so many organs and in so many conditions.

A consideration of the protean occurrence of the pigment in man reveals that although in some states in which it is found, a generalized nutritional imbalance might be suspected (*i.e.* malabsorptive states), in others such as atheroma, such imbalance is not, at least, so obvious. But a concept has now emerged which may serve as a useful working hypothesis to explain its presence in this wide variety of apparently unrelated conditions.

The concensus is that the pigment results from oxidation and peroxidation of polyunsaturated fats with the formation of long-chain polymers of an insoluble nature (K. M. Endicott, *Arch. Path.* **37**, *49* (1944); J. D. deOlivera, *Ann. N. Y. Acad. Sci.*, **52**, *125* (1949–50); G. M. Hass, *Arch. Path.* **26**, *1196* (1938); H. Dam and H. Granados, *Science* **103**, *327* (1945). Lillie, *Stain Technol.* **27**, *37* (1952)). Protein or amino acids have been found incorporated within it by some (deOlivera, *loc. cit.* P. György, *Am. J. Clin. Path.* **14**, *67* (1944)), but in other instances relatively pure forms consisting of only altered lipid have been reported (Endicott, *loc. cit.;* W. G. R. Casselman, *J. Exp. Med.* **94**, *549* (1951)). Probably it can present as a variable mixture of substances (C. S. Lee, *J. Nat. Cancer Inst.* **11**, *339* (1950)), but the polymerized unsaturated fat is the cardinal constituent.

It is quite clear that oxygen itself and substances which stimulate oxidation both *in vitro* and *in vivo* (Hartroft, *Science* **113**, *673* (1951)) may regularly initiate polymerization of the lipid. Saturated lipids are not involved, and the greater the degree of polyunsaturation, the more readily can ceroid be derived. Casselman (*loc. cit.*) demonstrated these principles in a series of rather elegantly devised experiments *in vitro*. Tocopherol and other antioxidants will, in a variety of situations, decrease formation of the pigment, even in the presence of rather abundant deposits of abnormal fat (A. L. Tappel, *Arch. Biochem. Biophys.* **54**, *266* (1955)). Oxidative catalysts, on the other hand, including hematin compounds, hemoglobin, cytochrome-C, and hemin, will favour its formation.

Hemoglobin itself is probably the most important single catalyst for its *in vivo* formation from polyunsaturated lipid accumulations, as indicated by simple experiments in which hemorrhage into the epididymal fat pad of normal rats or into fatty cysts of choline deficient rat livers is sufficient to stimulate abundant deposits of ceroid (Hartroft, *Am. J. Path.* **31**, *381* (1955)). It is likely that red blood cells act as the important catalyst in the pathogenesis of ceroid deposits in human atheromatous plaques (Hartroft, *J. Gerontol.* **8**, *158* (1953)).

It is apparent then that the nutritional status of the entire organism may play an important role in whether or not ceroid will be deposited in any part of the body. A high intake of polyunsaturated fat or a low intake of vitamin E, (and particularly the simultaneous presence of both conditions) will favor its formation, particularly if abnormal deposits of lipid form in liver, muscle, or other organs. But even in the case of an animal or man whose nutritional status might be regarded as essentially normal, it can be seen that focal lesions may precipitate a local condition which will favor the deposition of ceroid pigment. Any abnormality that results in the accumulation of excess amounts of lipid (usually stainable) nearly always implies at least some increase in polyunsaturated fat as well as saturated. If, in addition, there is coexistent hemorrhage, the latter acts as an ideal catalyst (by virtue of oxygen and hematin released from the degenerating erythrocytes) for the copolymerization of the unsaturated fat.

A useful working hypothesis can be summarized as follows: the greater the ratio of polyunsaturated to saturated fat at the site of any local accumulation of lipid, and the greater the ratio of oxidative catalysts to tissue antioxidants at the same site, the more abundant will be the formation of ceroid pigment. Such a coexistence of factors will more likely occur in the animal fed large amounts of polyunsaturated fats and low amounts of tocopherols, but the conditions necessary for ceroid formation can obviously exist locally (*i.e.* hemorrhage within a fatty liver or a fatty atheromatous plaque) without postulating any general nutritional abnormality.

The above concept can be expressed in the form of an equation:

$$\text{Ratio of } \frac{\text{Polyunsaturated fat}}{\text{Saturated fat}}$$

$$\times \text{ ratio of } \frac{\text{Oxidative catalysts}}{\text{Tissue antioxidant}}$$

$$= \text{Amount of Ceroid}$$

An example of the application of the principles embodied in the above formula, is afforded by experiments with choline deficient rats (Hartroft, *Am. J. Path.* **31**, *381 (1955)*). When they were fed such a diet, in which the fat was chiefly derived from lard (saturated), and generous supplements of tocopherol were given twice weekly by mouth, ceroid formation was almost entirely suppressed in the cirrhotic livers: but when corn oil was substituted for the lard and vitamin E was removed from the basal diet pair fed to other rats, ceroid was found in large amounts throughout every cirrhotic liver. Even in normal rats, crushing of the epididymal fat pad, producing mixtures of fat and red blood cells within the tissue, apparently releases enough polyunsaturated fat in a form which can intermingle with extravasated red cells to satisfy the conditions of the above equation so that ceroid is readily formed, as originally postulated.

The usual histochemical test for ceroid consists of carrying out an Oil red O stain on paraffin sections (from which all normal fat has been removed by their processing in alcohol and xylol). Using this test, ceroid has not always been demonstrated at sites in which the above hypothesis would predict its presence. For example, one might expect to find it consistently in all thrombi as a result of mixing polyunsaturated fats derived from serum with degenerating erythrocytes in and between the fibrin and platelet skeleton. But examination of coronary arterial thrombi from approximately 100 cases of fatal myocardial infarction by staining paraffin sections with Oil red O, revealed the pigment in only about half the number. An analogy drawn from publications by paint chemists suggested to us a possible explanation for its inconsistent presence. Naïve though this analogy may be, we risk citing it.

The hardening of an oil paint (usually a polyunsaturated fat such as linseed oil) into a hydrocarbon-insoluble film when spread on a wall occurs under the catalytic action of atmospheric oxygen and heat. Oils which undergo this reaction to completeness are termed "drying oils." But a number which are only relatively polyunsaturated (such as olive oil) will not harden no matter how long exposed to air and are termed "semi-drying oils." Such "semi-dried" oils are insoluble only in mild lipid solvents such as alcohol, but can be dissolved by stronger ones such as turpentine, xylol, or ether. This analogy suggests that within tissues also there could be a form of partially polymerized fats which, although not capable of resisting extraction with xylol (commonly used in preparing paraffin sections), would not be dissolved by alcohol in strengths barely adequate to remove normal, unaltered tissue lipids.

Using the crushed epididymal fat pad model, we were able to test this hypothesis (Hartroft, *Fed. Proc.* **22**, *250* *(1963)*). During the first week after operation and to a lesser extent subsequently, most of the altered lipid in the sections proved to be insoluble in 90 per cent ethyl or isopropyl alcohol (15 minutes extraction at 37°C.) but could be readily extracted with xylol (overnight at 37°C.). The milder extraction with alcohol was still sufficient to remove the unaltered fat within undamaged adipose tissue cells in the same sections. This semi-insoluble pigment, we called *interceroid* or *preceroid*. Examination of a series of tissues from man and experimental animals for the presence of this intermediate form has not yet been completed. It is possible that interceroid may be found in some of the conditions where ceroid was absent, although predicted to be present by our working hypothesis.

In conclusion, the notions expressed here would indicate that the formation of ceroid or interceroid may be a fundamental reaction of tissues to a wide variety of injuries both mechanically and nutritionally induced. The implications of this concept may have more than theoretical interest. It is likely that in some situations it is fibrogenic. It may have other effects as well. For example, we have recently been able to show that, when clots containing polyunsaturated fats are injected into the ear veins of rabbits, ceroid is subsequently formed after they are entrapped in the pulmonic vessels. The clots resisted fibrinolysis to a greater degree than was the case for control preparations similarly injected but which contained equal amounts of saturated fat (D. A. Legge and R. A. Bear, *Fed. Proc.* **25**, *324* *(1966)*; Bear, Legge, and Hartroft, *Ibid.* **25**, *324* *(1966)*).

The experiment was stimulated by the hypothesis that fibrin coated with ceroid in thrombi would not be readily accessible to the action of fibrinolytic enzymes and the results appeared to support it. If dietary polyunsaturated fat can be similarly incorporated in thrombi formed in man, one might postulate on this basis an increased resistance to thrombolysis with high oral intakes of vegetable fat. The implication in terms of current notions about dietary prophylaxis of myocardial infarction is obvious, but needs more exploration. We only cite this possibility (even if remote) to underline the need for further study of the entire problem of ceroid and interceroid by the pathologist, biochemist, and nutritionist alike in a multidisciplinary attack.

Chapter IX

PRESENT KNOWLEDGE OF NUTRITION IN RELATION TO DIABETES MELLITUS

Robert E. Hodges, M.D.

Although the precise incidence of the disease is not known, diabetes mellitus is found in all nations and peoples of the world. Reasonable estimates place the number of recognized diabetics in the United States at about two million persons, and perhaps another one and one-half million who have undiagnosed diabetes. Thus a crude estimate might place the figure at 2 per cent of the entire population of this country. This does not include the large group of people who have "latent diabetes" on a basis of an abnormal cortisone-glucose tolerance test. Experience has shown that at least one-fourth of all persons who are truly obese have latent diabetes and a surprisingly large segment of all elderly persons have abnormal glucose tolerance (*Nutrition Reviews* **20**, *192* (*1962*)). If all of these are included in a single group, diabetics recognized and unrecognized, latent diabetics with or without obesity, and elderly persons with an abnormal glucose tolerance curve, the total probably exceeds 10 per cent of the population of the United States.

Statistics indicate that an abnormal glucose tolerance test places people in a group subject to a greater than normal mortality rate. The death rate for persons with frank diabetes mellitus indicates that women are more adversely affected than men. In the non-diabetic white population the overall mortality at all ages is 10.5 per 1,000 persons per year compared with 11.4 for diabetic men. Non-diabetic women, on the other hand, have a mortality rate of only 6.4 per 1,000 per year compared with more than twice that rate, 13.6, for diabetic women. Thus the diagnosis of diabetes mellitus not only places a patient in a higher risk group, but also completely eliminates the sex differential which women customarily enjoy (*Statistical Bulletin* **45**, *7*, *August 1964;* **46**, *1, August 1965*).

If one examines the cause of death of diabetic patients it becomes apparent that vascular disease in general is excessively common and coronary heart disease in particular is far more common than it is in the general population. According to A. Marble (*Med. World News* **6** (*38*), *146* (*1965*)) the death rate from vascular disease in diabetics is two and one-half times greater than average for men and three and one-half times greater for women, but especially important is the early age at which death occurs from vascular disease. In persons from ages 15 to 34 diabetic men have 12 times the mortality rate and women almost 20 times the rate of non-diabetic populations.

We must ask ourselves whether this excessive mortality from vascular disease represents an inherent part of the diabetic trait, or a result of the manner in which we treat diabetes mellitus, or a combination of both these factors. Although we shall not be able to answer that question specifically, we can gain some insight into the problem by examining the available information.

We know, for example, that men hospitalized in this country with an acute myocardial infarction often will be found to have an abnormal glucose tolerance test at the time of their hospitalization. Re-examination of these persons a year later will disclose that approximately one-third of the total still have an abnormal glucose tolerance test; in other words they have either frank or latent diabetes. This suggests that the factor of inheritance may be a strong one, and that carbohydrate intolerance may be linked in some as yet undetermined manner to the atherosclerotic process. On the other hand, there are numerous reports which suggest that dietary practices may influence the incidence of clinically recognizable diabetes mellitus (J. Yudkin, *Lancet* **1**, *645* (*1956*); **2**, *155* (*1957*); **2**, *4* (*1964*); A. M. Cohen, *Am. Heart J.* **65**, *291* (*1963*)). Comparisons of the rate of mortality from diabetes in war and peace, or studies of the national consumption of certain foodstuffs as compared with the death rate from diabetes, do suggest that dietary factors influence the incidence of diabetes mellitus in its recognizable form.

During the past decade a great deal of research has been devoted to studies designed to relate the atherosclerotic process to dietary factors which might then be corrected. Certain disease states characterized by elevations of serum cholesterol and other lipids have been shown to be associated with a high incidence of ischemic heart disease (M. M. Gertler and P. D. White, *Coronary Heart Disease in Young Adults. Harvard University Press, Cambridge, 1954*; L. N. Katz and J. Stamler, *Experimental Atherosclerosis. Charles C Thomas Co., Springfield, Illinois, 1953*). Many investigators have reported a higher incidence of coronary heart disease among populations with high blood cholesterol levels than among populations with lower levels. One study (A. Kagan, W. B. Kannel, T. R. Dawber, and N. Revotski, *Ann. N. Y. Acad. Sci.* **97**, *883* (*1963*)) statistically links groups of people who have high serum cholesterol with a high incidence of coronary heart disease. Similarly, the concentration of triglycerides in the blood seems to be higher among groups with a greater coronary risk (M. J. Albrink and E. B. Man, *Arch. Int. Med.* **103**, *4* (*1959*)), although the supporting evidence is not as firm on this point. There can be no doubt about the ability of clinicians to lower the concentration of cholesterol in the blood of most patients by one of several dietary methods. In general, these methods include reduction of the amount of dietary cholesterol and substitution of unsaturated fatty acids for saturated ones, particularly myristic and palmitic acids (D. M. Hegsted, R. B. McGandy, M. L. Myers, and F. J. Stare, *Am. J. Clin. Nutrition* **17**, *281* (*1965*)). Preliminary evidence now suggests that lowering of blood lipid concentrations by dietary means may successfully lessen the incidence of coronary occlusion (G. J. Christakis *et al.*, *Am. J. Pub. Health* **56**, *299* (*1966*)).

Traditionally, patients with diabetes mellitus have been treated by dietary means. Before insulin became available the ketogenic diet not only reduced polyuria and polydipsia but in some cases was truly lifesaving (F. M. Allen, E. Stillman, and R. Fitz, *Rockefeller Institute Monograph 11. New York, 1919*). This diet was high in fats and proteins of animal origin and restricted intake of sugars and starches as much as possible. With the introduction of insulin the classical diet prescribed for the diabetic patient was modified cautiously to permit more carbohydrate, not only to please the patient's appetite but also to prevent ketosis. Usually 100 g. of carbohydrate per day is considered adequate for the latter purpose. Most diets recommended for diabetic patients still limit the carbohydrate allowance, often to less than 200 g. per day. Greater amounts than this have been avoided because of two beliefs: that more insulin would be required if more carbohydrate was fed and that substitution of carbohydrate for fat would lead to hypertriglyceridemia. Both of these opinions are now subject to review.

Meanwhile, the fate of diabetic patients in Japan appears to be of considerable interest (S. Wada *et al.*, *Diabetes* **13**, *485* (*1964*)). Although diabetes is at least as common in Japan as it is in the United

States the dietary management is entirely different. The Japanese patient with diabetes mellitus has few changes made in his customary menu aside from regulation of calories. He is allowed approximately 350 g. of carbohydrate daily and he eats only about 30 g. of fat daily. This is a result of custom and not of experimental design. It is interesting to note that the death rate of diabetic patients in Japan is considerably lower than it is in the United States: 9.3 per 1,000 per year for men and 10.5 per 1,000 per year for women (compared with 11.4 and 13.6 respectively in the U. S.). The frequency of vascular complications in diabetics appears to be lower in Japan than it is in the United States (T. Saito *et al.*, *Tohoku J. Exp. Med.* **71**, *87* (*1959*)) *i.e.*, less peripheral vascular disease, gangrene of the lower extremities, and coronary heart disease. Furthermore, acidosis is about one-tenth as common in these patients. Of course the question which must be asked is whether this difference in the apparent severity of the disease is a result of racial characteristics or of dietary habits. A comparison between carefully matched diabetic patients living in Japan with similar diabetic Japanese living in America would be highly enlightening.

Meanwhile there is good evidence to suggest that American diabetics can consume a diet which is chemically rather similar to that of the Japanese without either of the feared complications arising. D. B. Stone and W. E. Connor (*Diabetes* **12**, *127* (*1963*)) have compared the clinical and laboratory findings in diabetic patients who were given the traditional American Diabetes Association diet or an experimental diet which replaces large amounts of fats with carbohydrates. The experimental diet also markedly reduces the amount of cholesterol in the diet and the characteristics of the fat are changed to increase the degree of unsaturation. In the traditional diet about 100 g. of fat were fed, compared with 49 g. in the experimental, whereas 220 g. of

carbohydrate were replaced by 358 g. The usual 800 to 1,000 mg. cholesterol intake was reduced to 100 mg. daily. With this type of diet, diabetic patients were found to remain in good control and to require no more insulin than formerly. The concentration of both cholesterol and triglycerides in the blood decreased to a significant extent.

Other studies designed to evaluate the relationship between the diabetic diet and vascular complications are in progress in various parts of the world. Thus J. K. Lloyd is studying diabetic children who have been given diets containing considerably more polyunsaturated fat to replace the saturated fat in their diet (*Program of the Nutrition Society, Royal Infirmary, Edinburgh, October 30, 1965*).

In all the speculation regarding the possible role of diet in the high incidence of vascular disease in diabetic patients, one must not lose sight of the fact that they have the same nutritional requirements as anyone else. Children need ample amounts of high quality protein accompanied by sufficient calories and a proper supply of all the other essentials in the diet to insure proper growth and development. Adult diabetic patients must be ensured the same basic nutritional factors required by non-diabetics. The view that vitamin requirements may be higher in diabetics lacks firm support. Any controversy relating to the advantages and disadvantages of more or less carbohydrate or fat is secondary to these principles.

There are well-known nutritionists who still cling to recommendations of high fat diets for treatment of diabetic patients. Thus the most recent issue of a popular handbook states "concentrated sources of quickly absorbable carbohydrates, like sugar, candy, and fruit juices, are avoided and pure refined starches are limited as much as possible." (B. R. Burton, *The Heinz Handbook of Nutrition, Second Edition, p. 248. McGraw-Hill Book Co., Blakiston Division, New York, 1965*).

One report indicates that diabetics in China are fed a diet containing 338 g. carbohydrate, 38 g. fat, and 47 g. protein. These patients have lipid levels which are far lower than those of diabetic patients in the United States (but higher than non-diabetic Chinese) (Chung Hsueh-Li, Lin Shan-yen, Li Wen-Ching, and Ch'iu Ch'uan-lu, *Chinese Med. J.* **84,** *451* (*1965*)). The authors claim that "Under this diet, though the incidence of arteriosclerosis was higher in the diabetics than in the non-diabetic groups of comparable age and sex, it was lower than in many other countries and the disease was less severe." Although there seems to be no proof of this statement, perhaps the most encouraging aspect of the entire problem lies in the burgeoning degree of interest shown by investigators both in the Orient and in Western countries. Carefully designed studies can be anticipated to provide substantial information regarding the most favorable form of dietary management of diabetic patients.

Chapter X

PRESENT KNOWLEDGE OF NUTRITION AND DENTAL CARIES

James H. Shaw, Ph.D.

The past decade has provided much valuable information about the etiology of dental caries and the epidemiologist's triad of agent, host, and environment. No laboratory or clinical evaluation has complete validity today unless the investigator has ample guarantees that all three of these major etiological factors have been considered and controlled in the experimental design and procedures. Progress in this decade has been made primarily with studies on experimental animals; contributions from human studies have been minor except for those pertaining to fluoride, described in another review. Many findings made with experimental animals have yet to be adequately tested in clinical trials.

Dental caries in experimental animals occurs only in the presence of a suitable oral flora. Beyond any reasonable doubt, dental caries is of bacterial origin in man also. This necessity for microorganisms in experimental caries was first shown by F. J. Orland et al., (J. Dent. Res. 33, 147 (1954)) and confirmed by R. J. Fitzgerald, H. J. Jordan, and H. R. Stanley (Ibid. 39, 923 (1960)). Both groups maintained rats on caries producing diets under germfree conditions and saw no carious lesions.

Potentially caries-producing microorganisms appear to be much more limited in number than was believed a decade ago. It has been demonstrated under certain laboratory conditions that microorganisms responsible for caries production can be transmitted from one animal with active lesions to animals of the same species with no previous evidence of caries activity. Continuation studies with parallel procedures led to the recognition that five biochemically similar strains of streptococci isolated from a carious lesion in a hamster were individually capable of producing carious lesions in caries-inactive hamsters (Nutrition Reviews 19, 105 (1961)). Pooled cultures of six strains of diphtheroid organisms, or six strains of lactobacilli isolated from caries-inactive hamsters were ineffective when similarly inoculated. An interesting finding, not adequately explained or explored, indicated that there was very little cross-susceptibility of the hamster to rat microorganisms, and vice versa (R. J. Fitzgerald, Ibid. 66, 597 (1963)).

K. S. Berman and R. J. Gibbons (Arch. Oral Biol. (London) 11, 533 (1966)) studied the ability of various microorganisms to store intracellular iodophilic polysaccharide. Strains of streptococci capable of producing carious lesions in hamsters and rats were able to synthesize and store this type of polysaccharide, and then able to utilize it during the absence of an exogeneous energy source. The streptococci known to be inactive in producing carious lesions in animals were incapable of uniform production and storage of polysaccharide. In addition, 60 per cent of cultivable bacteria from human carious lesions were found to be strong polysaccharide producers, while only 13 per cent from caries-inactive plaques were strong producers.

Gibbons, Berman, P. Knoettner, and B. Kapsimalis (Arch. Oral Biol. (London) 11, 549 (1966)) observed that each of two strains of streptococci isolated from human carious lesions was able to cause extensive lesions in otherwise germfree rats. A third strain was not able to induce caries under similar circumstances. Seven rodent and human cariogenic streptococci have been found to form large quantities of extracellular non-dialyzable capsules from carbohydrates like sucrose, suggesting that capsule formation may be important in the carious process, enabling the microorganisms to adhere to tooth surfaces.

In another type of study, D. D. Zinner, J. M. Jablon, A. P. Aran, and M. S. Saslaw (*Proc. Soc. Exp. Biol. Med.* **118,** *766* (*1965*) ; *Proceedings of Forty-third General Meeting, International Association for Dental Research, abstract 261* (*1965*)) isolated from human carious lesions microorganisms immunologically similar to strains isolated from oral cavities of rats and hamsters, and found that some of these strains would cause lesions in rats and hamsters.

Obviously, insufficient data are available as yet to draw broad generalizations. However, the possibility of a specific antibiotic(s) for depressing growth of microorganisms responsible for carious lesions in man is not nearly as remote as heretofore. Presently, little is known as to whether any nutrient in the diet will alter microbial flora directly.

Much less is known about the host factor than about bacterial agents or environmental influences of carbohydrates. Many epidemiological surveys of primitive populations have indicated a much lower prevalence of dental caries than in more highly developed societies (G. N. Davies, in *Caries-resistant Teeth, G. E. W. Wolstenholme and M. O'Connor, Editors. Little, Brown and Co., Boston* (*1965*)). The tendency has been to interpret these findings as indicative of high caries resistance of genetic origin. Little attention has been paid to the possibility that in primitive societies food patterns may have contributed nutrients during tooth development that influenced caries susceptibility after development was complete.

Probably, in many primitive populations there has not been an adequate challenge, either bacterial or oral environmental, or both. Indeed, determinations of whether populations or specific individuals are caries-resistant genetically, because of nutrition during tooth development, or simply inadequately challenged by simultaneous bacterial and oral environmental routes, are almost impossible to make at our present level of knowledge. The Indian population has been considered for decades to be caries resistant genetically. However, J. M. Dunning and J. H. Shaw (in *Nutrition and Caries Prevention, G. Blix, Editor. Swedish Nutrition Foundation, Stockholm, 1965*) discuss several variables, such as high fluoride levels in the enamel and dentin of Indian teeth, infrequency of eating, inadequate caloric supplies, low availability of monosaccharides and disaccharides, and a high degree of sunshine throughout the year, all of which could act to keep caries incidence low, quite apart from genetic constitution.

Possibly individuals who remain caries free for prolonged periods in areas where caries prevalence is high may be better examples of resistance than primitive populations. Numerous investigators have selected caries free individuals from such large populations as subjects. In general, these studies have provided little evidence of any single factor responsible for this low caries index. Yet even these individuals may never have been adequately challenged.

In animal studies, strains of rodents have been selected to emphasize characteristics of caries resistance or susceptibility. The Hunt-Hoppert strains are best known. In the resistant strain, dental caries did not develop under experimental conditions until about 600 days of age, on the average, whereas lesions were present in the susceptible offspring by 70 days.

When resistant or susceptible rats were nursed by mothers of the opposite strain from birth, the caries scores remained typical of their genotypic inheritance. Likewise, when the oral flora of young rats was depressed by penicillin and then reestablished by inoculation from both strains, caries scores again were typical of the genetic background (S. Rosen et al., J. Dent. Res. **41**, *1013* (*1962*)). Similar studies with the Harvard resistant and susceptible strains indicated a tendency for offspring to exhibit phenotypic characteristics for caries prevalence typical of their genotypic constitution (Shaw, D. Griffiths, and A. Terborgh, *Arch. Oral Biol.* **7**, *693* (*1962*)).

Under other environmental circumstances, the Hunt-Hoppert strain demonstrated much higher levels of caries involvement than reported by Rosen *et al.* When the Harvard strains were tested under other bacterial challenges and dietary conditions, R. H. Larson (*J. Dent. Res.* **44**, *1402* (*1965*)) observed much higher caries attack rates than in the findings of Shaw and co-workers.

These studies indicated clearly that the relative intensity of the cariogenic challenge varied from laboratory to laboratory and that caries resistance and susceptibility were relative terms. A challenge suitable to elicit demonstrable differences between strains must be employed.

Probably the clearest evidence of a genetic factor was provided by Larson and M. E. Simms (*Science* **149**, *982* (*1965*)). Female rats of a white strain were double mated with males of the same strain and males of a black strain in which black is dominant. Homozygous white offspring had a much higher caries prevalence than the heterozygous black offspring. No experimental circumstances had provided a more similar dietary and bacterial challenge than this study. The only evident explanation for the difference between the offspring appears to be the chromosomal contribution of the fathers.

No conclusive evidence for other developmental influences—other than fluoride (*see* the chapter on Fluoride)—in human nutrition has been presented. However, in experimental animals other influences need brief comment.

Nutrition during tooth development has been shown to modify the teeth with respect to size, time of eruption, and later caries susceptibility. Earlier work has been reviewed by K. J. Paynter and R. M. Grainger (*J. Am. Med. Assn.* **177**, *306* (*1961*)). Borderline vitamin A deficiency, a low calcium-phosphorus ratio (1:3), or a supplement of 12 p.p.m. fluoride imposed on female rats throughout pregnancy and lactation resulted in smaller molars among the offspring. Under these experimental conditions, vitamin A deficiency did not affect the incidence of dental caries, while the low calcium-phosphorus ratio resulted in higher caries activity.

Later studies in rats with borderline protein deficiency throughout pregnancy and lactation caused smaller molars among offspring, later eruption of the molars, higher dental caries incidence, and missing cusps on the third molars (Shaw and Griffiths, *J. Nutrition* **80**, *123* (*1963*)). Since the protein deficiency was mediated through the mother, no final conclusion of the actual mechanism for causing these changes in the offspring can be made. As yet no evidence is available to indicate that protein deficiency during tooth development in man would have comparable effects.

In rats, supplements of sodium chloride, lithium carbonate, strontium carbonate, and ammonium paramolybdate resulted in significant increases in the offsprings' caries susceptibility (Shaw and Griffiths, *Arch. Oral Biol.* (*London*) **5**, *301* (*1961*)). Again these results are difficult to interpret because dietary supplements must be given the mother during pregnancy and lactation rather than directly to the offspring. B. J. Kruger (*J. Dent. Res.* **41**, *215* (*1962*)), by injection of boric acid, sodium fluoride, or ammonium molybdate into nursing rat pups between birth and 11 days of age, attempted to circumvent this problem. Caries susceptibility was reduced in all tests and resulted in sulci in the molars that were broader and shallower than those of the controls.

Many meticulous, carefully controlled experiments will be needed to find the answers in this area. In all probability one or more species of subhuman primates will be necessary for adequate investigation of relationships, not only to caries susceptibility, but also to chemical composition and morphology.

The whole environment is of paramount importance in the general level of dental caries incidence. Such parameters as quantity and type of available foods, dietary patterns, economic status, annual hours of sunshine, humidity, type and amount of clothing, composition of water supplies, and oral hygiene are determined by the environment and make a contribution to the level of caries in the population. More specifically, the oral and especially the micro-environment on the caries-susceptible tooth surface determines largely whether the surface will decay. When appropriate microorganisms with suitable nutrients are present, the likelihood of tooth decay is extremely high.

The pivotal food component is carbohydrate. In experimental rodents, many studies have reported high incidence of carious lesions when the diets contained monosaccharides and disaccharides, but greatly reduced incidences when only starches were present. Studies with man suggest that the same difference may be demonstrable. Dental surveys of Seventh Day Adventist children have indicated that they consistently have less tooth decay than children of other groups in the same community (R. A. Down, M. M. Dunn, and E. L. Richie, *Am. Assn. Pub. Health Dent. Bull.* **18**, *19* (*1958*); C. J. Donnelly, *Pub. Health Rep.* **76**, *209* (*1961*); R. L. Glass and J. Hayden, *J. Dent. Child.* **33**, *22* (*1966*)).

All authors credited the lower caries rate among the Adventist children to discouragement, as a religious precept, of eating sweets and between-meal snacks.

The effects of oral hygiene and sweet consumption were studied by J. N. Mainsbridge (*Brit. Dent. J.* **109**, *343* (*1960*)).

The 146 children in the 12 to 14 year old group who were considered to have good oral hygiene had a mean decayed, missing, and filled (DMF) tooth rate of 9.58 in contrast to 11.47 for the 118 children considered to have neglected their oral hygiene. This difference was significant at $p = 0.01$. When the amount of sweet and chocolate consumption was considered, the 177 children with less than eight ounces consumption per week had DMF values of 9.60 in contrast to 10.83 for those who had consumed more than eight ounces per week. This difference was also significant at $p = 0.01$.

The possibility that starches are not highly cariogenic in man has not been fully tested. However, evaluations of caries incidence in patients with fructose intolerance, who tend to omit all monosaccharides and disaccharides from their diets, have indicated much lower levels than in their normal relatives or the general population (E. R. Froesch *et al.*, *Am. J. Med.* **34**, *151* (*1963*); M. Cornblath *et al.*, *New Engl. J. Med.* **269**, *1271* (*1963*)).

B. Krasse (*Arch. Oral Biol.* **10**, *215*, *223* (*1965*)) has reported that sucrose was able to support a more rapid progression of carious lesions in the hamster than glucose. He drew attention to work by J. Carlsson and J. Egelberg (*Odont. Rev.* **16**, *42*, *112* (*1965*)), who reported greater accumulation of plaque in dogs and man when sucrose was present. In the rat little or no difference between sucrose, glucose, and maltose was observed (Shaw, I. Krumins, and R. J. Gibbons, *Arch. Oral Biol.* **12**, *755* (*1967*)).

An effect of phosphates on dental caries, largely during the post-developmental period, has received much attention. Under many circumstances, various inorganic and organic phosphates cause less dental caries in experimental rodents. In human populations, little or no benefit was observed (*Nutrition Reviews* **23**, *307* (*1965*)).

A post-developmental relationship between dental caries and pyridoxine has been suggested by several studies. There was a higher than usual incidence of caries in *Rhesus* monkeys fed pyridoxine deficient diets. Since this subhuman primate species rarely develops carious lesions in comparison with the commonly used rodent, the level of caries incidence described was considered to be striking. Studies with hamsters on cariogenic diets supplemented with additional amounts of pyridoxine have indicated modest benefits.

Twenty mg. pyridoxine were provided in a vitamin-mineral capsule or 20 mg. divided among 3 lozenges daily to two groups of women during pregnancy. The main difference between the groups appeared to be the number of women with no increase in caries during approximately 6 or 7 months, with 54 per cent remaining caries free in the lozenge group and only 32 per cent in a third control group. The average increase in dental caries for the women who developed new lesions was very similar for the three groups (*see Nutrition Reviews* **21**, *143, 145* (*1963*)).

These data are interesting because of their consistency rather than for any large highly significant reductions in dental caries incidence. If a real effect attributable to pyridoxine exists, it is impossible to say whether the action is upon oral microorganisms or human subject.

Whether protective factors occur naturally in foods is not known definitely. In laboratory studies with rodents, indications of the existence of such factors have been observed. The phytates, largely lost in milling grains, have been shown to be mildly antagonistic to the caries process (F. J.

McClure, *Science* **144**, *1337* (*1964*); C. Dawes and Shaw, *Arch. Oral Biol.* (*London*) **10**, *567* (*1965*)). F. Takita and P. H. Phillips observed that adding 10 per cent oat hulls to cariogenic diets reduced carious lesions in the cotton rat. Certain polyphenols with anti-caries activity were obtained by fractionation. Later, K. O. Madsen and E. J. Edmonds observed that the outer parts of other seeds such as rice, peanut, cottonseed, and pecan all caused reductions in dental caries (*see Nutrition Reviews* **21**, *244* (*1963*)).

In various *in vitro* tests, G. H. Jenkins (in *Nutrition and Caries Prevention*) studied the ability of various natural foods and their components to inhibit acid production and dissolution of calcium from tooth samples. He reported a high protective effect from raw cane juice and blackstrap molasses and believed that a complicated mixture of substances was responsible.

Detailed knowledge about the causes of caries has increased greatly with regard to microbial agents and the environment of the tooth, but much less with regard to the host. The best procedures for the control of dental caries include a well-balanced diet composed of a good variety of foodstuffs, fluoridation of public water supplies or the provision of an appropriate amount of fluoride through another source when fluoridation is not feasible, good oral hygiene, and the elimination of between-meal snacks composed largely of monosaccharides and disaccharides in forms that adhere readily to tooth surfaces and have a low oral clearance.

Chapter XI

EXPERIMENTAL ALCOHOLIC HEPATIC INJURY

W. Stanley Hartroft, M.D., Ph.D. and E. A. Porta, M.D.

The broad spectrum of hepatic lesions associated with prolonged consumption of alcohol in man ranges from the simple accumulation of neutral fat in hepatocytes to true monolobular and multilobular cirrhoses. Studies of serial liver biopsies now appear to indicate that all these lesions are stages of the same evolutionary process, and have also pointed to the frequency of multiform inflammatory and degenerative changes found in cirrhotic and non-cirrhotic alcoholics with acute hepatic insufficiency, long histories of heavy alcohol intake, recent drinking to excess, and poor food intake. By no means a separate morpho-pathologic entity, this "acute alcoholic hepatitis," as it has been termed, is the most characteristic and "florid" structural feature encountered in alcoholics. Recent electron microscopic studies have broadened the pathologic complex to include a wide variety of mitochondrial and endoplasmic reticular changes. Some details (controversially interpreted) in the configuration of Mallory bodies are almost pathognomonic of this condition.

The hepatic fatty changes are almost always encountered in biopsy specimens of those alcoholics recently admitted to hospital and before any extensive treatment is instituted. Fat droplets of various sizes are found within most hepatocytes, except in regenerating areas. These droplets often coalesce to form large globules that displace nuclei to one side. Fatty cysts of variable size are frequently encountered in these livers. Although some authors have questioned the hepatocytic nature of the wall of fatty cysts, electron microscopic studies have shown that in rats (W. S. Hartroft, in *Aktuelle Probleme der Hepatologie, G. A.*

Martini, Editor. Georg Thieme Verlag, Stuttgart, 1962) as well as in human alcoholics (E. A. Porta, B. J. Bergman, and A. A. Stein, *Am. J. Path.* **46,** *657* (*1965*)), the walls are indeed formed by hepatocytes (not Küpffer cells).

Occasionally, fatty cysts become entrapped within fibrous trabeculae, although most of the fat in this location is found within macrophages. Fat droplets are also present within Küpffer cells but are outnumbered by granules of ceroid present not only in these phagocytic cells but also in many trabecular macrophages in the livers of chronic alcoholics. Specimens taken from autopsy cases may eventually show absence of fat, but even in these cases the finding of intratrabecular fatty cysts and ceroid-containing macrophages will strongly suggest that the cirrhosis was at one time a fatty one.

Enlargement of mitochondria, which appears as the most conspicuous change in hepatocytes (with or without fat) of the alcoholic, includes elongation as well as spherulation or even more bizarre giant configurations (megamitochondria). Mitochondrial cristae are altered or absent and not infrequently matrical crystalline-like inclusions are found in these giant misshapen organelles.

Although in the opinion of C. Biava (*Lab. Invest.* **13,** *301* (*1964*)), Mallory bodies represent a unique lesion of the hepatocytic endoplasmic reticulum, histochemical and electron microscopic evidence indicates that they represent degenerated *megamitochondria*. Furthermore, for the first time this peculiar alcoholic hyaline body can now be reproduced in experimental animals chronically consuming alcohol (*vide infra*) and its origin traced at the ultrastructural levels (Porta, Hartroft, and F. de la Iglesia, *Lab. Invest.* **14,** *1437* (*1965*)). The paranuclear acidophilic bodies encountered in paraffin sections of hepatocytes of rats fed several alcoholic liquid diets displayed the same tinctorial affinities which characterized Mallory bodies found in human alcoholics (E. E. Minaker and Porta, *J. Microscopie* **6,** *41* (*1967*)). The ergastoplasm of hepatocytes may degenerate, if either the commonly seen vesiculation and disaggregation of ribosomes or the more commonly found hyperplasia and reorientation of the lamella of smooth and endoplasmic reticulum associated with parallel and concentric rows of glycogen granules could be interpreted as such. The endoplasmic reticulum probably bears little demonstrable relation to the origin of Mallory bodies.

Should the alcohol per se be considered as an hepatotoxin able to produce these structural and ultrastructural hepatic alterations, described above, in its full range? Controversial views abound, since a cause and effect relation has not yet been clearly established. The fact that only a small fraction of alcoholics develop cirrhosis would suggest that the effect of alcohol is probably not that of a direct hepatotoxin in the usual sense.

In this regard, A. Y. Olsen (*Am. J. Med. Sci.* **220,** *477* (*1950*)), obtained dietary histories indicative of protein deficiency in 45 per cent of cirrhotic alcoholics at the Los Angeles County Hospital. High protein intake even without withdrawal of alcohol improves the hepatic lesions of chronic alcoholics (W. Volwiler, C. M. Jones, and T. B. Mallory, *Gastroenterology* **11,** *164* (*1948*)). Furthermore, Reynolds *et al.* have recently shown the beneficial effect of large doses of alcohol (up to 440 ml. per day ethanol) to patients hospitalized with "decompensated" alcoholic cirrhosis and given a daily protein intake of 55 to 75 g. (*Symposium on Therapeutic Agents and the Liver, N. McIntyre and S. Sherlock, Editors, p. 131. Blackwell*

Sci. Pub., Oxford, 1965). Dietary anomalies (not necessarily nutritional deficiencies but possibly dietary imbalances or a combination) are almost certainly frequently implicated, at least as important contributing factors in the etiology. Since a chronic alcoholic may easily consume more than 2,000 calories per day in the form of alcohol, it is obvious that when this many calories are superimposed on an even relatively well balanced solid diet (let alone one which is low in protein to begin with) imbalances must almost certainly be precipitated. Dietary surveys in alcoholics have sometimes neglected this aspect.

One of the most interesting studies on the food habits of the alcoholic is that of W. G. Figueroa *et al.* (*Am. J. Clin. Nutrition* **1,** *179* (*1953*)), who screened large numbers of alcoholics admitted to the House of Correction of Chicago. They found that obtaining a reliable dietary history from an alcoholic was extremely difficult if not impossible. A formal history proved quite unreliable, but more precise information was obtained by engaging various alcoholic inmates in conversation and then offhandedly discussing their consumption of food and alcohol. To evaluate further the dietary intake of these men, several field observations were made in the "Skid Row" of Chicago. On this basis it was estimated that the average daily consumption of protein was only about 30 g. per day. It was postulated that a considerable number of underweight (and probably some of the euweight) alcoholics were suffering from depletion of protein. A large proportion of the diet was made up by carbohydrates, since the alcoholics ate quantities of bread and doughnuts, sandwiches, and spaghetti. These authors did not calculate the proportions of calories from fat, carbohydrate, protein, and alcohol, but the imbalance is obvious.

Clinicians, faced with persistent consumption of alcohol in their patients, should perhaps in each instance carefully evaluate the pattern of total calories consumed (alcohol plus food) to make sure that the solid portions of their diets are supplying sufficient of all food factors, especially protein, to give as nearly balanced a ration *in toto* as possible, taking into account the large number of "empty" calories provided by the liquor.

A second question is pertinent here: Can alcohol injure the human liver if the diet is truly adequate in every respect? Any answer at the present state of our knowledge is bound to be controversial. But information gathered from acute and chronic experiments in rats has permitted elucidation of some aspects of the chemical defect in lipid metabolism induced by alcohol. However, in the opinion of the current authors, a major gap in experimental hepatology still exists in that all attempts to reproduce in experimental animals the complex, multifaceted type of lesion encountered in chronic human alcoholics have still failed even after years of effort by many.

Some progress toward the goal has perhaps been made by duplicating Mallory bodies in rats consuming large proportions of alcohol (36 per cent of total caloric intake) mixed with relatively high fat (43 per cent) and adequate levels of protein-16 per cent-diets (*loc. cit.*). But due perhaps to the relatively short duration of the experiments (12 weeks), or more likely other factors still unknown, cirrhosis was not produced. Because Mallory bodies have been infrequently reported in the absence of cirrhosis in man it is of interest that they were encountered in great numbers in these rats' livers. The hepatic fatty changes, which are almost universally found in livers of human alcoholics, are readily induced in animals consuming alcohol. These changes precede, as in human beings, all other structural and ultrastructural changes, even in the acute model.

Acute and chronic experimental models differ in several significant aspects, including the nature and lobular localization of lesions as well as the response of the liver in

each case to dietary supplements. Oral administration of ethanol at the mildly intoxicating dose currently used in the acute model promptly results in transient accumulation of lipids (almost exclusively triglycerides) in *periportal* hepatocytes. The fat is deposited as tiny droplets that rarely coalesce to form bigger globules, which do not displace nuclei. The laden hepatocytes are not appreciably enlarged. These fatty changes are followed by other transient ultrastructural alterations such as enlargement and coalescence of mitochondria, endoplasmic reticular disarrangement, hyperplasia of Golgi complex, and depletion of glycogen.

Isocaloric amounts of sucrose also induce to a lesser degree an accumulation of fatty droplets in periportal hepatocytes, but the cytoplasmic ultrastructural configuration of the cells remains unaltered. The acute ethanol induced fatty liver is not modified by simultaneous oral administration of choline, but is prevented by antioxidants (vitamin E and G-50), as demonstrated by N. R. Di Luzio (*Am. J. Physiol.* **194,** *453 (1958);* *Life Sci.* **3,** *113 (1964)*) and recently confirmed (Hartroft, Porta, and M. Suzuki, *Quart. J. Stud. Alcohol* **25,** *427 (1964);* Porta and Hartroft, in *Symposium on Therapeutic Agents and the Liver, p. 145*). The high levels of blood alcohol achieved by this procedure and consequently the sudden influx of alcohol into liver cells may create enzymatic disturbances, responsible in turn for profound metabolic disorders. In this sense the injury to the liver produced by alcohol in this model could be termed a toxic action.

Conversely, in chronic experiments in which the daily intake of alcohol is fourfold or fivefold that employed in the acute model, the conditions approximate more closely those found in human alcoholics. The greater amount of alcohol is consumed more slowly over many hours in both instances. Although early effects of the chronic situation are also manifested by accumulation of abnormal amounts of triglyceride in hepatocytes, the liver fat is found *centrolobularly* instead of *peripherally* as in the acute. Localization of fat in liver lobules may reflect the influence of other factors in the diet rather than any peculiarity of chronic alcohol consumption per se. In this regard, current long-term experiments involving dietary manipulations of the caloric proportions of fat, protein, and carbohydrates indicate that the lobular location of fat does not depend on alcohol which otherwise is kept constant (36 per cent), but on imbalances of several other dietary constituents (Porta, Hartroft, de la Iglesia, and Gomez-Dunn, *Am. J. Path.* **48,** *39a (1966)*).

The use of alcohol-containing liquid diets introduced by C. S. Lieber, D. D. Jones, J. Mendelson, and L. M. DeCarli (*Tr. Assn. Am. Phys.* **76,** *289 (1963)*) permits fine control, not only of any dietary constituent, but also the amount of alcohol consumed, which can under these conditions be elevated much higher than in experiments in which solid diets were employed and the alcohol administered in the drinking water. Young animals given the alcoholic-food liquid mixture grew relatively well (3 g. per day) and usually equalled growth of controls, which were pair fed isocaloric diets in which sucrose replaced alcohol. In livers of rats which consumed alcohol, fat droplets appeared in the cytoplasm of hepatocytes within one week and became progressively larger. But even after 12 weeks, formation may have been averted because sufficient protein (16 per cent of total calories) was provided in these diets to enable proliferation of enough new liver cells to accommodate the abnormal lipid load in intracellular form, thereby avoiding cell rupture and consequent cyst formation. In support of this notion, in rats of other experiments in which the protein was kept at a low level (6 per cent calories), fatty cysts were found within four weeks (Hartroft *et al.*, *Gastroenterology* **50,** *392 (1966)*).

In all these chronic experiments the most conspicuous ultrastructural changes affect mitochondria. Early elongation of these organelles proceeds to tortuous and branching configurations. Monstrous mitochondria frequently encircle portions of cytoplasm, other small mitochondria, and particularly droplets of fat. Bizarre mitochondria often cohere and clump. By the second week, megamitochondria are sometimes even bigger than nuclei. Once they had attained such a size it was obvious that it should be possible to observe them by light microscopy. And so indeed they are observable, and so indeed have they been noted for more than a quarter of a century—because they are the well known and familiar Mallory bodies of alcoholism. With the exception of crystalline-like material in the matrix of mitochondria of human alcoholics, all the ultrastructural cytoplasmic alterations found in hepatocytes of these patients have now been duplicated in these animals.

Dietary vitamin E supplements given to rats which were chronically consuming liquid diets containing alcohol, a high amount of fat, and an adequate level of protein, neither modified the amount of lobular deposition of triglycerides as in the acute model (*vide supra*) nor prevented the ultrastructural changes of the hepatocytes.

Experiments in rats recently reported by D. P. Jones (*Am. J. Clin. Nutrition* **16,** *381 (1965)*) indicate further the implications of dietary imbalances in the pathogenesis of alcoholic fatty liver. It seems now that alcohol consumed along with normal (relatively low fat, normal protein) diets does not induce significant degrees of hepatic fatty change. In this situation, certainly alcohol cannot be regarded as hepatotoxic. More recent chronic experiments in rats consuming relatively high amounts of alcohol and "super diets" high in protein and excessive in vitamins and lipotropes showed that all the hepatic alterations were effectively prevented (O. R. Koch, Porta, and Hartroft, *Lab. Invest.* **16,** *629 (1967)*). Furthermore, administration of these "super diets" to cirrhotic rats permitted the functional and morphologic recovery of hepatic alterations even in the presence of high alcohol consumption (A. Takada, Porta, and Hartroft, *Am. J. Clin. Nutrition* **20,** *213* (*1967*)).

These reviewers, who have struggled for some years to unravel the complex pathogenesis of alcoholic hepatic injury, now feel somewhat humble. The "retrospectroscope" indicates rather clearly that the hepatic lesions seen in human alcoholics are most likely neither a toxic effect of this nectar nor the consequence of a deficiency of a single vitamin or essential food factor. The history of clinical nutrition contains numerous examples of the failure of surveys of any population or group to disclose the existence of disease in man produced in a pure form associated with a single deficiency. Almost without exception a complex of several has been found, whether the subjects were Eskimos or Belsen inmates.

In alcoholics, we already know that the neuritis which may afflict these unfortunates can be prevented or corrected by administration of Vitamin B_1. It is now well established that there are a number of food factors, the lack of which is first manifested in the liver. Choline, methionine, selenium, vitamin E, and essential fatty acids are outstanding in this regard, to mention only a few. Alcohol calories are "empty" when superimposed in large numbers on even a "perfect" diet, which then of course can only provide a fraction of the total calories consumed. Important deficiencies are almost certain to develop and manifest themselves in an appropriate organ (liver, nerve, or heart) sooner or later. We (and others) have been guilty in the past of focusing on our "favourite vitamin" and forgetting that in the alcoholic as in the pregnant woman or even normal man, the principles of sound nutrition can never be disregarded.

Chapter XII

PRESENT KNOWLEDGE OF NATURALLY OCCURRING TOXICANTS IN FOODS

Olaf Mickelsen, Ph.D.

Selectively toxic substances

Some naturally occurring substances may be innocuous by themselves but under certain conditions may cause toxic manifestations. An example is tyramine in such foods as aged cheddar cheese, Chianti, and yeast extracts. Tyramine toxicity becomes manifest only in patients receiving an inhibitor of monoamine oxidase, who then develop acute hypertension, palpitation, and flushing. In a few, the attack may be so severe that death results.

If ingestion of the mushroom *Coprinus atramentarius,* or inky-cap, is followed by consumption of an alcoholic beverage, the face of the drinker, and perhaps other parts of his body, soon becomes purplish-red (J. M. Kingsburg, *Poisonous Plants of the United States and Canada, p. 26. Prentice-Hall, Inc., Englewood Cliffs, New Jersey, 1964*). Interaction of alcohol and the mushroom produces a compound related to the action of antabuse.

Celiac disease has been associated with the gluten fraction of wheat, which produces toxicity symptoms in those few individuals who are allergic to this substance. There was a marked increase in celiac disease among Dutch infants during World War II when wheat temporarily became the primary dietary staple (*Nutrition Reviews* 21, 195 (1963)).

Vitamin-related toxic substances

Some essential nutrients may be toxic when consumed in excessive amounts. The margin of safety varies considerably for the nutrients and, perhaps, among individuals. While the possible toxic effects of vitamins A and D are discussed elsewhere in this volume, it should be noted that there appears to be an antagonism of vitamin A to vitamin D toxicity (*Nutrition Reviews* 20, 315 (1962)). In rats the toxic effects of large doses of vitamin D could be overcome by equally large or larger doses of vitamin A (on the basis of I.U.). These studies are of interest, since symptoms of vitamin D toxicity are best treated by removing it from the diet. Can the recovery period be shortened and the patient experience a better recovery if large amounts of vitamin A are given?

Thiaminase in certain foods is in the category of naturally occurring toxic substances. This enzyme splits the thiamine molecule between the pyrimidine and thiazole groups. Since higher animals cannot recombine these two groups, a thiamine deficiency results.

Pyridoxine deficiency in chicks fed flaxseed meal has been shown by H. J. Klosterman and co-workers to be due to a naturally occurring antagonist (*for review, see* O. Mickelsen and M. G. Yang, *Fed. Proc.* 25, 104 (1966)). This is one of the first such compounds to be isolated from natural products. The potency of the pyridoxine antagonist is equal to that of 4-deoxypyridoxine for chicks and a thousand times more active for *Azotobacter.*

Dicumarol may be related to the antagonists. First isolated from "spoiled" sweet clover hay, it inhibits formation of prothrombin and is formed by oxidation of coumarin to 4-hydroxycoumarin during spoilage. Subsequently, two molecules of the latter compound condense with formaldehyde. The hemorrhagic condition associated with ingestion of dicoumarol can be overcome or prevented in most animals by vitamin K. For man, naturally occurring vitamin K appears more active than 2-methyl-1,4-naphthoquinone in counteracting an overdose of dicoumarol.

Toxic substances that interfere with mineral metabolism

Oxalic acid, which inhibits efficient calcium utilization, occurs in fairly high concentrations in Swiss chard, spinach, lamb's quarters, beet tops, marigolds, halogeton (goosefoot plant), sorrel, purslane, and rhubarb. In halogeton, it approaches 37 per cent of the dry weight of the leaves. Introduced into Nevada about 1930, the plant spread to most of the surrounding semi-arid regions, and was presumably responsible for the deaths of large numbers of sheep. Among techniques developed to counteract the toxicity is feeding alfalfa pellets containing 15 per cent calcium carbonate when animals graze in heavily infested areas.

Recent work has shown that iron absorption is reduced by a protein-like substance present in certain species of raw fish (*Nutrition Reviews* **19**, *143* (*1961*)).

The phytates in a variety of plants have interfered with absorption of many minerals. One of these deficiencies of considerable practical importance is parakeratosis in swine (*Nutrition Reviews* **15**, *334* (*1957*)). The condition could be largely overcome by addition of extra zinc to the soybean meal ration. In chicks fed sesame meal (*Ibid.* **19**, *111* (*1961*)), zinc deficiency occurred despite adequate zinc in the ration and use of galvanized cages and watering troughs.

The toxic action of goitrogens in a variety of compounds can be overcome by addition of extra iodine to the ration. These substances have produced enlarged thyroids in rabbits fed oats, hay, and fresh cabbage. For experimental animals, a variety of plants, including rapeseed, black and white mustardseed, Brussels sprouts, cauliflower, kohlrabi, and soybeans have been reported to be goitrogens.

The activity of these goitrogens varies from one species to the next. Propylthiouracil is 11 times more potent than thiouracil in the rat and only three-fourths as active in man. To determine which goitrogens may be toxic for man, a technique has been developed to permit rapid evaluation of a food. By such means, M. A. Greer and his associates showed that rutabaga had the highest goitrogenic activity. They isolated a goitrogen (2-hydroxy, 3-butenyl isothiocyanate) which exists in the plant as progoitrin. The latter is converted to the active substance, goitrin, by an enzyme, myrosinase (Greer, *Rec. Adv. Endocrinol.* **18**, *187* (*1962*)).

Although many attempts have been made to relate the presence of endemic goiter to use of goitrogenic food in various parts of the world, there is little evidence for such a relationship either in man or in animals. Even the possible transmission of goitrogens through milk of cattle fed plants with considerable amounts of goitrin poses no health problem (A. I. Virtanen, M. Kreula, and M. Kiesvaara. *Z. f. Ernaehrungswiss. Suppl.* **3**, *23* (*1963*)).

Toxic substances in legumes

1. *Peas.* Spastic paralysis, especially of the legs, is one of the earliest symptoms of lathyrism in human subjects (A. L. Weaver and J. A. Spittell, Jr., *Proc. Mayo Clin.* **39**, *485* (*1964*)) who have consumed large amounts of *Lathyrus sativus*, *L. cicera*, or *L. clymenum*. These plants survive periods of drought; consequently, in countries such as India, there is an increased incidence of the disease during famines, when as much as 7 per cent of the population may be afflicted (*Nutrition Reviews* **25**, *231* (*1967*)).

Although horses and cattle are reported to develop paralysis in those areas where lathyrism is endemic, the rat appears to be highly resistant. Absence of a condition in laboratory animals analogous to lathyrism in man has hindered isolation of the factor responsible. However, D. N. Roy, V. Nagarajan, and C. Gopalan (*Current Sci.* **32,** *117 (1963)*) have reported neurological disturbances in chicks injected with an alcoholic extract of *L. sativus*.

L. odoratus, the common sweet pea, in contrast, is highly toxic to rats. The toxicity has been duplicated by two compounds related to the beta-(N-gamma-L-glutamyl)-aminopropionitrile originally isolated from *L. pusillus* (singletary pea). Subsequent work showed that beta-aminopropionitrile and aminoacetonitrile were the active substances.

Whereas the toxic factor in *L. sativus* affects the human nervous system, the two nitrile compounds interfere with collagen formation. The nitriles may produce their effect by inhibiting incorporation of sulfate, glucose, and glycine into chondroitin sulfate (M. J. Karnovsky and M. L. Karnovsky, *J. Exp. Med.* **113,** *381 (1961)*).

2. *Faba beans.* Inhalation of the pollen or ingestion of *Vicia faba,* cooked or raw, produces, by an unknown mechanism, a hemolytic anemia in individuals with a deficiency of glucose-6-phosphate dehydrogenase and, as a result, a reduction in glutathione blood levels (W. H. Zinkham, R. E. Lenhard, Jr., and B. Childs, *Bull. Johns Hopkins Hosp.* **102,** *169 (1958)*). Ingestion of *faba* beans still further reduces glutathione content of the red cells, and this is associated with hemolysis of the older cells. Since younger red cells resist hemolysis, patients usually recover once the severe hemolysis has ceased (E. Beutler, in *The Metabolic Basis of Inherited Disease, J. B. Stanbury, J. B. Wyngaarden, and D. S. Fredrickson, Editors. McGraw-Hill, New York, 1960*).

In some areas of the world (the Mediterranean, Asia, or Formosa) the sensitivity to *faba* or broad beans affects a fair proportion of the people. Yet on Formosa, the Joint Commission on Rural Reconstruction supports cultivation of *faba* beans as a dietary staple and a green fertilizer (J.-Y. Lin and K.-H. Ling, *J. Formosan Med. Assn.* **61,** *484 (1962)*). The toxic substance in *faba* beans has not yet been isolated.

3. *Soybeans.* Toxic substances in the raw beans have been studied extensively. Ruminants, especially after their microflora has been established, appear relatively insensitive to the toxic factors. Although all young monogastric animals show various abnormalities (primarily poor growth) when fed raw soybeans, the chick appears to outgrow this difficulty, and heating the beans improves growth.

It was early observed that addition of cystine to the raw soybean ration also improved growth, but the original suggestion that heating made the cystine and methionine in the raw beans more available has been complicated by more recent work (*for discussion, see* Mickelsen and Yang, *loc. cit.*). It is very likely that the growth inhibition associated with ingestion of raw soybeans is attributable to a number of factors (*Nutrition Reviews* **23,** *346 (1965)*). A recent report suggests that the raw bean may produce a systemic disturbance involving methionine metabolism (*Ibid., loc. cit.*).

Despite the number of toxic factors in raw soybeans, none of these appears to have any effect when the meal is properly toasted. The high biological value of properly prepared soybean meal is one reason why its production in the United States has increased so rapidly (W. W. Cravens and E. Sipos, in *Processed Plant Protein Foodstuffs, A. M. Altschul, Editor., p. 353. Academic Press, New York, 1958*).

4. *Other beans.* In the raw state, kidney, navy, lima, or pinto beans contain toxic substances, most of which are heat labile. Feeding uncooked navy beans to rats not only inhibits growth but produces acinar atrophy of the pancreas, fatty degeneration of the liver, follicular atrophy of the thyroid, and hyperkeratosis of the esophagus and skin. Attempts to isolate the toxic sub-

stance resulted in separation of the growth depressing and hemagglutinating properties (*Nutrition Reviews* **24**, *121* (*1966*); M. L. Kakade and R. J. Evans, *Brit. J. Nutrition* **19**, *269* (*1965*)).

Toxic substances in cottonseeds

Toxicity of raw cottonseed meal involves primarily gossypol, and, to a much lesser extent, sterculic acid. Calves, guinea pigs, rabbits, swine, and dogs, roughly in that order, appear to be susceptible to gossypol toxicity, rats and poultry much less so.

Sterculic acid in cottonseed oil produces a pink color in the whites of eggs laid by hens fed the oil or meals containing small amounts. Until recently, the color change was primarily of economic importance, but a report suggests that sterculic acid and related fats may interfere with reproduction in rats and chickens (A. M. Roscop, E. T. Sheehan, and A. R. Kemmerer, *Proc. Soc. Exp. Biol. Med.* **122**, *142* (*1966*)).

Mushrooms

There is a great deal of variability reported in the toxicity of the same species of mushrooms. This stems from: (1) Problems in classification, as with *Amanita*, some of the most poisonous. (2) Sensitivity can develop: some species (*Gyromitra esculenta*) that resemble morels can be eaten for the first time without any untoward effects, but the second time produce symptoms of toxicity. (3) Conditions under which, and the geographic area where mushrooms are grown. (4) For many mushrooms, the toxic principle is destroyed or inactivated when the plants are dried or cooked. (5) Individual predilection, with some people able to eat mushrooms with impunity, while others develop severe toxicity when eating the same kind. (6) The extent to which the mushrooms have been processed prior to eating and the amount consumed.

Toxic substances in mushrooms vary in chemical structure and symptoms produced.

Some toxic compounds in the *Amanita* are polypeptides, which contain various substituent groups. For some, antisera have been produced which are reported effective if given shortly after symptoms develop. Other mushrooms contain a number of alkaloids; the best known is muscarine, a derivative of choline. Although muscarine has been isolated from a number of species, there is little evidence that it is responsible for the syndromes produced by ingesting these plants (Kingsbury, *Op. cit., p. 90*).

Symptoms of toxicity vary both with the species and with the individual. In many cases, vomiting occurs and thus reduces the amount of toxin absorbed. Thereafter, the patient may develop severe abdominal pain, prostration, and jaundice. For some species, such as *Amanita muscaria*, symptoms of poisoning are highly characteristic. Increased activity of the salivary, lacrymal, and sweat glands appears within one-half to three hours. Copious watery diarrhea, auditory and visual hallucinations, cardiac inhibition, and gastrointestinal tract stimulation also occur. The hallucinatory properties of this mushroom account for its use by the natives in some parts of Eastern Russia (Kingsbury, *Op. cit., p. 94*).

Other toxins, such as those from *Amanita phalloides*, cyclopeptides with a thioamide structure, presumably act on cell membranes. The symptoms include severe abdominal pain, nausea, and vomiting ten to 20 hours after eating, followed by delirium and occasionally convulsions which may go on to collapse and stupor. Toxic substances in *A. phalloides* are thermostable. Although an antiserum has been reported for these compounds, its efficacy remains to be established (A. Grollman, *Pharmacology and Therapeutics, p. 338. Lea and Febiger, Philadelphia, 1962*).

Death is certain with only a few species, and most of these involve *A. phalloides* or their close relatives. Thirty-five deaths in the United States from 1924 to 1961 were attributable to eating mushrooms. When unreported or undetected cases are added to this, the number is probably doubled.

Molds

Diseases caused by molds have been grouped under the term mycotoxicoses. Ergotism is one of the oldest. It has long been associated with flour prepared from grain on which the mold *Claviceps purpurae* has grown. Symptoms have been reported after eating bread made with flour in which as little as 1 per cent came from contaminated grain (*Nutrition Reviews* **20,** *237 (1962)*). A number of pharmacologically active compounds have been isolated from the ergot fungi which mimic the symptoms seen in ergot poisoning. Although ergot poisoning is popularly associated with abortion, this does not occur unless fairly large amounts ("dangerous doses") of the active compounds are consumed for long periods.

The importance of mycotoxicoses among animals was emphasized by a number of recent epidemics traceable to these plant forms. One that aroused a great deal of interest and research was traced to peanuts on which a variety of *Aspergillus flavus* (*Link*) grew (*Nutrition Reviews* **20,** *174 (1962)*; **22,** *97 (1964)*). A number of crystalline compounds were isolated from the mold cultures. Four have been characterized, principally on the basis of physical data, and called aflatoxins (T. Asao *et al., J. Am. Chem. Soc.* **85,** *1706 (1963)*; **87,** *882 (1965)*).

These molds and their toxic substances appear to be ubiquitous. They contaminate peanuts and cottonseed meal, and perhaps yams and corn (*Nutrition Reviews* **20,** *339 (1962)*; **22,** *62, 208 (1964)*). A number of other disease conditions in farm animals have been related to the presence of molds in food, forage, or litter. One of these is hyperkeratosis in cattle, which initially was attributed to a chlorinated hydrocarbon. Some reports suggest that a bread mold (*Aspergillus chevalieri*) might be implicated.

A hemorrhagic disease which affected large numbers of commercial laying hens may have been caused by a variety of molds. At least some that were isolated from infected hen houses were reported able to produce the syndrome when incorporated into chicken feed (*Nutrition Reviews* **20,** *339 (1964)*).

Chapter XIII

PRESENT KNOWLEDGE OF VITAMIN A

Oswald A. Roels, Ph.D.

Man's earliest knowledge of vitamin A was a deduction from symptoms of disease caused by its absence. Night blindness, a marked impairment of vision at low light intensity, has troubled man for thousands of years. It is undoubtedly for this reason that the visual process was of first interest in the study of vitamin A.

With the work of G .Wald (*Vitamins and Hormones* **18,** *417* (*1960*)) and R. A. Morton (*Nature* **153,** *69* (*1944*)) and others, much progress has been made in our understanding of this role of vitamin A. The retina of most vertebrates contains two distinct photoreceptor systems. The rods are especially sensitive to light of low intensity; the cones receive high light intensities and colors. Retinal is the prosthetic group of photosensitive pigments of the rods in land vertebrates and in marine fish, 3-dehydroretinal in fresh water fish.

The biochemial mechanism of cone vision is analogous to that of rod vision; photoreceptors of both systems contain identically the same chromophore—either retinal or 3-dehydro-retinal, depending upon the animal species. The protein moiety of these systems is not the same in rods as in cones, so that the major difference between the visual pigments in each is the protein bound to the chromophore.

Biochemical reactions involved in the oxidation of retinol to retinal, and stereochemical changes in the side chain of the vitamin A molecule which occur in the visual process, have been studied in detail. All-*trans* retinol is oxidized to all-*trans*-retinal; this compound isomerizes to the 11-*cis* form which, combined with opsin, forms rhodopsin. After absorbing light quanta the 11-*cis* isomer of retinal or of 3-dehydro-retinal is converted to the corresponding all-*trans* form.

Energy to operate this reaction against a potential gradient is supplied by the light quanta. This energy exchange causes potential differences, which produce a nervous excitation transmitted via the optic nerves to the brain, resulting in visual sensations. The potential difference caused by the breakdown of rhodopsin when it absorbs light can be measured by an electroretinograph. This measurement can then be used to assess the vitamin A status of animals and man.

Absorption, transport, and storage of vitamin A in mammals also have been studied extensively.

In most mammals, the product ultimately absorbed from the intestinal tract after feeding provitamins A is vitamin A itself. There is, however, a great deal of species specificity in the ability of different mammals to absorb dietary carotenoids. Man and the bovines can absorb both vitamin A and the carotenoids, and convert carotenoids with provitamin A activity to the vitamin. In constrast, the rat and the pig do not absorb significant amounts of carotenoid pigments. However, they have the ability to convert provitamins A to the vitamin. Although the small intestine is the most important organ involved, other tissues are also capable of carrying out this process. It has recently been demonstrated that perfusion of isolated rat liver with ^{14}C-labeled beta-carotene produces labeled retinyl ester (*Nutrition Reviews* **21,** *238* (*1963*)).

A number of factors affect absorption of the provitamins A from the intestine. The level of dietary fat is important in man's absorption of carotenoids. Fat represents less than 7 per cent of the total caloric intake in Ruanda and Urundi (Central Africa), and, although the diet there contains an ample supply of carotenoids, these are so inefficiently absorbed that vitamin A deficiency appears frequently in young boys. Small fat supplements markedly improve carotenoid absorption from the intestine in these boys, increase serum vitamin A levels, and alleviate symptoms of the deficiency.

Conjugated bile acids with one free hydroxyl group have a stimulating effect on carotene absorption and on cleavage of the carotene molecule in intestines of chicks, hamsters, rats, and rabbits. Low protein diets reduce intestinal absorption of vitamin A and its esters.

Absorption and transport of vitamin A can be summarized as follows: dietary retinyl ester is hydrolyzed in the lumen of the intestine before passage across the mucosal cell wall. Retinol, from dietary sources or resulting from the hydrolysis of dietary retinyl ester, passes the mucosal cell wall, and is reesterified inside the cell, preferentially with palmitic acid. Retinyl palmitate in chylomicrons travels through the lymphatic system, via the thoracic duct, to the blood stream, and is stored in the liver. Stored retinyl ester is hydrolyzed there by a liver enzyme; free retinol then travels via the blood stream to the tissues where a metabolic requirement exists. Retinol is mobilized from the liver and its level in blood is maintained, even on a diet without vitamin A, until all liver reserves are exhausted.

Like most other lipids, vitamin A and the provitamins A are transported in body fluids in the lipoprotein form. Retinyl ester occurs mainly in the Sf 10–100 lipoprotein fraction of the blood stream. Twenty per cent of the free retinol present in serum is associated with the Sf 3–9 serum lipoprotein fraction, which also carries about 80 per cent of the beta-carotene and lycopene in human serum. Since retinyl ester is transported from

gut to blood stream in the chylomicrons (Sf > 400), the half life of the newly absorbed retinyl ester in chylomicrons must be short.

However, retinal, retinol, and retinyl ester are not the only active forms. All-*trans*-retinal has about 90 per cent as much activity outside the visual cycle as all-*trans*-retinyl-acetate. The bio-potency of retinal outside the visual cycle seems to depend entirely upon its enzymatic reduction to retinol: many animal tissues contain an enzyme capable of this reduction. In 1946, D. A. Van Dorp and J. F. Arens (*Rec. Trav. Chim.* **65**, *338* (*1946*)) synthesized retinoic acid and demonstrated that this form can support growth of vitamin A deficient rats. When retinoic acid is fed to young rats on a diet lacking other forms of the vitamin, they grow normally but soon become night blind, eventually go completely blind, and cannot reproduce. It seems likely that retinoic acid is transformed into other compounds which may be "active" forms of vitamin A, and may play an essential role in animal metabolism.

A derivative of retinoic acid, possibly the glucuronide, has recently been discovered in the enterohepatic circulation of the rat. Synthesis of retinal epoxide with biological activity has also been reported.

The search for a general function of vitamin A outside the retina first centered on the possibility that it plays a role in keratinization, cornification, and mucus formation. It seems to be necessary for the formation of mucus secreting cells, which synthesize glycoproteins, and contain mucopolysaccharides. In vitamin A deficiency keratinization is more pronounced and formation of these cells is depressed.

Keratinization is required for formation of inert structural components of the body. Bone changes in vitamin A deficiency or in hypervitaminosis A were found to be associated with changes in chondroitin sulfate. All these observations point towards a possible role of the vitamin in mucoprotein synthesis and perhaps in synthesis of the mucopolysaccharide moiety of the mucoprotein molecule. Controversial claims have been made about the vitamin's effect on the incorporation of sulfate into mucopolysaccharides and on the activation of sulfate to form 3'-phospho-adenosine-5'-phospho-sulfate.

An increased urinary excretion of inorganic sulfate has been observed in rats deficient in vitamin A. Sulfurylation of paranitrophenol by rat liver supernatant is also reduced in vitamin A deficiency. However, recent reports of markedly increased lysosomal sulfatase activity in livers of rats deficient in vitamin A, coupled with an increased release of acid hydrolases from the liver lysosomes, suggest that the apparent reduction in sulfate incorporation might be due to increased sulfatase activity. Vitamin A may well play a role in polysaccharide metabolism, but since synthesis and degradation occur simultaneously, the net result will depend on the relative rates of the two processes.

E. Mellanby's observation that hypervitaminosis A caused bone and nerve lesions in animals (*J. Physiol.* **101**, *408* (*1942–1943*)) was followed by tissue culture studies, which indicated that addition of fairly large doses of vitamin A to the medium caused cessation of growth, followed by disintegration of the bone cartilage (*see Nutrition Reviews* **10**, *343* (*1952*)). H. B. Fell and co-workers found later that an excess of vitamin A added to the medium dissolved the chrondroitin sulfate in cartilage. This effect was shown to be due to rupture of lysosomal membranes, followed by release of acid hydrolases from lysosomes into the medium. These hydrolases then caused tissue disintegration (*see Nutrition Reviews* **20**, *161* (*1962*)).

The same effect has been observed in different species, and recent work has shown that liver lysosomes of rats deficient in vitamin A also become very labile. Normal vitamin A concentration ensures optimum stability, but large doses labilize the lysosomal membrane *in vivo*, as well as *in vitro*. This effect plays a role in many different membrane systems, such as the erythrocyte outer membrane and the mitochondrial membrane.

In carbohydrate metabolism, it was found that vitamin A deficiency did not disturb the tricarboxylic acid cycle. However, glycogen biosynthesis from acetate, lactate, and glycerol appears to be slowed down and can be reversed by cortisone administration.

Interaction between the vitamin A group of compounds and other members of the lipid class has also been studied extensively. Vitamin A metabolism is linked with that of coenzyme Q, vitamin E, vitamin D, the sterols, and the biosynthesis of squalene. Interaction of vitamins A and E seems to be important in regulating stability of biological membranes (O. A. Roels, M. Trout, and A. Guha, *Biochem. J.* **97**, *353* (*1965*)). Morton and his collaborators found that ubiquinone (coenzyme Q) increased in the liver of vitamin A deficient rats (*see Nutrition Reviews* **19**, *218* (*1961*)). Vitamin A deficiency increases synthesis of squalene and ubiquinone in rat liver and reduces cholesterol synthesis.

It has been shown that utilization of liver vitamin A stores is directly proportional to protein intake when animals are fed a diet low in the vitamin. Low protein diets retard the onset of deficiency symptoms.

Several studies have indicated that vitamin A influences synthesis of both serum and muscle proteins. Whether this effect is direct or indirect remains to be seen.

Protein malnutrition and vitamin A deficiency are probably the two most common nutritional deficiency diseases in the world today. Frequently both occur simultaneously, often with fatal results.

Patients with kwashiorkor often have very low serum vitamin A levels. When adequate dietary proteins are given, levels rise without administration of vitamin A, provided there are sufficient liver reserves. The implications are of the utmost importance to the nutrition of children in areas where there is a high incidence of kwashiorkor and vitamin A status is marginal. Since a skim milk supplement is frequently used in kwashiorkor treatment, and results in an increased vitamin A requirement, it may mobilize the last reserves from the liver, and thus precipitate vitamin A deficiency. This is not an argument against feeding a high grade protein to children with kwashiorkor, but emphasizes the need for a vitamin A supplement as well.

An excess of vitamin A may also have a very serious effect on man and animals. The acute form of vitamin A intoxication has been noted in persons ingesting excessively high single doses, or large quantities of polar bear liver. Chronic hypervitaminosis A occurs in patients who receive large doses for dermatologic conditions and continue subsequent intake without medical supervision. Severe cases of hypervitaminosis A have been encountered in faddists who include excessively large doses of vitamins in their daily diet.

A wide variety of signs and symptoms may appear. Fatigue, malaise, and lethargy are common complaints, frequently accompanied by one or more of the following symptoms: abdominal discomfort, bone and/or joint pain, severe throbbing headaches, insomnia and restlessness, night sweats, loss of body hair, brittle nails. Other symptoms may be exophthalmus, peripheral edema, yellow waxy pigmentation of the soles, palms, and nasolabial folds due to carotenoid deposits. Increased intracranial pressure and increased cerebral spinal fluid pressure have been observed. Hydrocephalus and lowered CSF pressure have been reported in calves with hypervitaminosis A.

The most serious public health problem related to this vitamin, however, is still its deficiency. The seriousness and clinical consequences, mainly in young boys throughout the world, have been emphasized in a recently published report (H. A. Oomen, D. S. McLaren, and U. Escapini, *Trop. Geograph. Med.* **16**, *271* (*1964*)). The authors conclude that xerophthalmia remains a major health problem in many parts of the world, especially in rapidly growing urban centers of the East like Hong Kong, Djakarta, Manila, Saigon, and Dacca.

Xerophthalmia is a major cause of blindness in childhood, yet vitamin A deficiency is often the result of ignorance. Rich sources of provitamin A are frequently available at little or no cost to families in areas where the deficiency is prevalent. Therefore, nutrition education can play an important role in eradicating this disease. The protective effect of a large depot dose of vitamin A should be investigated. It is possible to administer a single large dose intramuscularly, intravenously, or orally, and obtain good liver storage. This protects the child for a relatively long period from the disastrous results of an inadequate dietary supply.

Vitamin A palmitate now sells for approximately five U.S cents for 1,000,000 I. U. Since the daily requirement of an adult human is about 3,000 I. U., it is apparent that to provide the entire annual requirement of one human being would cost about five U.S. cents. It is truly amazing, in view of this, that vitamin A deficiency remains one of the most widespread forms of human malnutrition, with its untold consequences of social and individual misery.

Chapter XIV

PRESENT KNOWLEDGE OF THIAMINE

Michael C. Latham, M.B., M.P.H., D.T.M. & H.

The synthesis of thiamine and the elucidation of its structure were achieved by R. R. Williams and J. K. Kline (*J. Am. Chem. Soc.* **59**, *1504* (*1936*)). Thiamine hydrochloride was found to be a compound consisting of a pyrimidine ring joined by a methylene bridge to a peculiar thiazole nucleus. The composition is $C_{12} H_{18} N_4 OSCl_2$ with the following chemical structure:

The bond between the two rings is weak, with the result that the compound is easily destroyed, particularly in an alkaline medium. It is the only compound produced by living matter which has a thiazole ring.

Thiamine hydrochloride occurs in spicular crystals. It is highly soluble in water and thus easily leached out of foodstuffs being washed or boiled.

An important stage in the breakdown of glucose is the formation of pyruvic acid which, in the absence of oxygen, is reduced to lactic acid. During exercise lactic acid accumulates in the muscles and passes into the body fluids. With a supply of oxygen the lactic acid is oxidized back to pyruvic acid. The pyruvic acid undergoes oxidative decarboxylation, forming acetyl-CoA, which enters the tricarboxylic acid cycle (the Krebs cycle).

What is of interest to nutritionists is that thiamine is part of the coenzyme responsible for this decarboxylation. Thiamine is necessary in the diet for the formation of co-

carboxylase. Without cocarboxylase, pyruvic acid accumulates in various tissues. Thiamine must be phosphorylated before it can act as a coenzyme. Cocarboxylase, which is in fact thiamine pyrophosphate, acts with diphosphopyridine nucleotide (which contains nicotinic acid), coenzyme A (which contains pantothenic acid), and lipoic acid to oxidatively decarboxylate pyruvic acid to acetyl coenzyme A.

Another function of thiamine pyrophosphate is the oxidative decarboxylation of alpha-ketoglutaric acid. Thiamine pyrophosphate is also the coenzyme in the transketolase reaction.

Thiamine may be assayed using chemical, biological, biochemical, and microbiological means. The early methods were biological, using pigeons, chickens, rats, and sometimes other animals. Microbiological assays have used *Phycomyces blakesleeanus* or *Lactobacillus fermentum*. Other workers have used the yeast fermentation procedure. However, the most widely used assay techniques are various modification of the thiochrome method. These involve oxidation of thiamine to thiochrome, which is then measured with the fluoroscope or by a colorimetric procedure. The method is fairly accurate and not very time-consuming.

H. Baker, O. Frank, J. J. Fennelly, and C. M. Leevy (*Am. J. Clin. Nutrition* **14**, *197* (*1965*)) recently suggested use of the protozoan flagellate *Ochromonas danica*. It has a sensitive and specific thiamine requirement and has been used as a reagent for thiamine determinations in blood, serum, cerebrospinal fluid, urine, muscle, and liver tissue. The method yields qualitative results in two days and quantitative results in five days.

More controversial than the assay method of choice is the selection of a means to detect early or marginal thiamine deficiency in man. Measurement of blood levels of thiamine and thiamine pyrophosphate is of limited value, for even when clinical manifestations of beriberi are present there is only a slight reduction in these values. It has been suggested that total blood thiamine levels below 3.0 μg. per 100 ml. in the absence of anemia should be regarded as indicative of a thiamine deficiency state.

Thiamine deficiency leads to an elevation of pyruvic acid in the blood. Blood pyruvate levels have therefore been used as a test for thiamine deficiency (W. N. Pearson, *Am. J. Clin. Nutrition* **11,** *462* (*1962*)). M. K. Horwitt and O. Kreisler (*J. Nutrition* **37,** *411* (*1949*)) concluded that the study of blood lactate and pyruvate in mild deficiency has little diagnostic value. They devised a test that measured lactic and pyruvic acids after glucose administration and exercise.

Pearson states that at the present time the most useful biochemical index of thiamine intakes in human population groups is measurement of urinary excretion of thiamine, usually expressed as excretion of thiamine per gram of creatinine. The ICNND has, during its surveys in many countries, produced a large body of data and has suggested interpretative standards for adults. There is a need for good standards for children.

Although urinary thiamine levels may be useful in nutrition surveys, this is not a reliable test of thiamine deficiency in the individual patient. Urinary levels fall relatively soon after the dietary intake is reduced and well before there is a tissue depletion of the vitamin. The kidney has no threshold for retaining thiamine, so that even loading tests are not reliable. Thiamine given intravenously, even in a person with thiamine deficiency, will tend to spill over into the urine.

A specific relationship between thiamine nutriture and transketolase activity at the enzyme or cellular level in man (M. Brin, *Am. J. Clin. Nutrition* **12,** *107* (*1963*)) has led to development of a new test using erythrocytes. The advantage of using an easily obtained tissue such as the red blood cell is obvious. Brin postulates that two subjects may have very different levels of thiamine in the tissue or urine, yet both may have adequate vitamin for enzyme activity. It is only when the enzymes have inadequate vitamin cofactors that tissue metabolism suffers. Erythrocyte transketolase activity may be useful in evaluating thiamine adequacy for normal cellular metabolism.

In a recent study, excretion of thiamine and its metabolites has been measured in the urine of men receiving restricted intakes (Z. Z. Ziporin *et al., J. Nutrition* **85,** *287* (*1965*)). These workers found a very rapid decrease in thiamine excretion. They consider that thiamine in the urine is "spillover" thiamine not utilized by the body, and that it does not accurately reflect body stores. It is, however, not associated with a similar lowering of the excretion of the pyrimidine moiety of thiamine. Metabolites excreted in the urine may be viewed as indicators of utilized thiamine, whereas the transketolase assay measures the amount of thiamine in the blood and is related to the amount in such tissues as liver, kidney, and muscle. Thus, while both measure the vitamin in different media or tissues, each indicates different aspects of thiamine status.

A recent attempt to assess human thiamine requirements has been made (Ziporin *et al., loc. cit.*) by measuring the thiamine metabolites in the urine of adult males on a restricted intake. These workers believe that when thiamine in the urine is no longer detectable, metabolites appearing in the urine are an index of the amount of thiamine taken from the tissue stores and utilized for metabolic needs. They calculate that the thiamine requirement is 0.27 mg. or 0.33 mg. per 1,000 calories, depending on whether the small amount ingested by their subjects is or is not subtracted from the metabolite output. This work has not yet been repeated in women or children.

It has been demonstrated, in laboratory animals and man, that the dietary requirement for thiamine varies with the composition of the diet. Carbohydrate is particularly important, and a diet providing most of its calories from fat results in thiamine sparing. This may result from a lowered metabolic requirement for thiamine if energy is derived from nutrients other than carbohydrate. It does not, however, explain the thiamine sparing action of certain carbohydrates and of antibiotics.

For example, rats develop evidence of thiamine deficiency earlier when the carbohydrate used is glucose or sucrose rather than potato starch. The requirement for thiamine is also reduced when sulfonamides, penicillin, and similar antibiotics are in the diet. Such findings have led to investigation of intestinal microflora as a possible additional source of thiamine. It is suggested that antibiotics, for example, cause a relative suppression of some, and a proliferation of other, microorganisms with resultant increased synthesis (or decreased diversion) of thiamine, and do not alter absorption or tissue utilization.

M. C. Nath and S. K. Meghal (*Biochem. J.* **81,** *220* (*1961*)) showed that protection from thiamine deficiency was possible when rats were fed thiamine deficient diets which support the growth of intestinal microorganisms. Dietary sucrose and glucose suppressed fecal coliform bacterial counts and failed to protect animals from thiamine deficiency. Meghal and Nath suggested that a drastic alteration of the lipid content of a diet may affect microbial vitamin production (*Brit. J. Nutrition* **19,** *189* (*1965*)). They concluded that a high fat diet enhances thiamine synthesis in the intestine of thiamine deficient rats and that the extent of this increase depends on the degree of saturation of the fat and the presence in it

of essential fatty acids. This increased synthesis is presumed to be associated with an increase in the population of microorganisms. There are therefore those who favor the microbiological as opposed to the metabolic explanation of the thiamine sparing action of fat.

The sparing action of some carbohydrate derivatives such as sorbitol (T. B. Morgan and J. Yudkin, *Vitamins and Hormones* **20,** *39* (*1962*)) and of antibiotics is probably the result of microbial synthesis of thiamine in the intestine, its excretion in the feces, and ingestion of feces by the rat. Prevention of coprophagy abolishes the sparing effect of penicillin (M. S. Mameesh, R. E. Webb, A. W. Norton, and B. C. Johnson, *J. Nutrition* **69,** *81* (*1959*)) and of sorbitol (Morgan and Yudkin, *Nature* **184,** *909* (*1959*)).

Yudkin (*J. Nutrition* **81,** *183* (*1963*)) has shown that rats given a thiamine free diet survived longer when kept directly on the floors of their cages where they had an easy access to their feces than when kept on grids. He concluded that most if not all the thiamine was available for absorption. Earlier work of B. S. Wostmann and P. L. Knight (*J. Nutrition* **74,** *103* (*1961*)) suggested little or no absorption of flora synthesized thiamine even following coprophagy in rats.

These authors used ^{35}S, and judged absorption by radiothiamine in hearts and muscles. They found that the main site of microbial synthesis was the cecum. The flora of the digestive tract was found to incorporate radiosulphate into the *in situ* formed thiamine molecule. Perhaps the rats in these experiments did not consume much of their own feces, or the thiamine obtained in this manner constituted a very small proportion of their total thiamine intake.

There is in certain uncooked fish an enzyme, thiaminase, capable of destroying thiamine. Human consumption of uncooked clams reduces availability of thiamine by approximately 50 per cent. Evidence is accumulating that thiaminases are widely distributed, being found in fish, ferns, bacteria, and related organisms. R. Hayashi (*see Nutrition Reviews* **15**, *65* (*1957*)) believes that the thiaminase of bacteria are not worthy of nutritional consideration except for certain "thiaminase bacteria" namely *B. thiaminolyticus, B. aneurinolyticus,* and *Cl. thiaminolyticus.* The action of thiaminase is to split the thiamine molecule into two parts, a pyrimidine and a thiazole moiety.

During the last decade there has been no major contribution to our knowledge of the disease beriberi. Both wet (cardiovascular) and dry (neuritic) beriberi have been attributed by some authors to a deficiency of several vitamins, but there is now fairly wide agreement that thiamine deficiency is the major factor. Adequate clinical descriptions of the disease including infantile beriberi are to be found in many textbooks of nutrition and internal medicine, and are not therefore appropriate here.

Beriberi became a scourge in the last century as the milling industry marched across Asia producing polished rice for poor people at a financial cost no more than that of home pounded rice, but at a cost of many thousands of lives. Highly refined, very white flours are rapidly becoming popular in many African countries (M. C. Latham, *Human Nutrition in Tropical Africa. FAO, Rome 1965*).

Some authorities feel that no real problem exists with corn. Yet highly milled corn flour as sold in much of East Africa has 0.05 mg. thiamine per 100 g. compared with 0.06 mg. thiamine per 100 g. in highly milled polished rice in endemic beriberi areas of the Far East. In highly milled corn meal the level of riboflavin is similar to that in rice, and the niacin content is lower. Seeing the danger ahead, some countries in Africa are contemplating legislation to ensure an adequate vitamin content of milled cereal flours (Latham, *Proceedings of Sixth International Congress of Nutrition, 449. Livingstone, Edinburgh, 1965*). It is obvious that enrichment of a cereal flour is a much simpler measure than the enrichment of rice, usually bought and cooked in its granular form. There is still no unanimity with regard to the best means of prevention of beriberi in rice eating areas. R. J. Williams (*Towards the Conquest of Beriberi. Harvard University Press, Cambridge, Mass., 1961*) has been a champion of pre-mix enrichment, whereas an FAO committee (*FAO Nutrition Studies No. 12, Rome, 1954*) have been very cautious in their recommendation.

Discussing nutrients available per capita per day in the U. S., Oris V. Wells (*see Nutrition Reviews* **17**, *161* (*1959*)) showed a figure of 1.79 mg. thiamine, including that added to prepared cereals, white flour, and bread. His data showed a fairly uniform supply of thiamine available from food to families in all income groups.

Industrial production of thiamine has increased greatly over the last few decades. The synthetic process usually involves separate synthesis of the thiazole and the pyrimidine halves of the molecule followed by its coupling. Apart from the demands of medical practice and the pharmaceutical trade, the food industry is now a large user of thiamine for fortification of many foods. There is also a tremendous prevalence of self-medication with vitamins. Physicians too tend to overprescribe thiamine, regarding it as a panacea for neurological aches and pains. In fact, the conditions in which thiamine plays a role are fairly limited. Fortunately, in the case of thiamine the body is very good at getting rid of the excess.

J. A. Campbell and A. B. Morrison (*Am. J. Clin. Nutrition* **12**, *162* (*1963*)) have indicated that the size of the dose significantly influences excretion. Oral doses above 2.5 mg. appear to be largely unabsorbed, and there is probably little justification for their use in vitamin therapy. Divided doses of thiamine are absorbed to a significantly greater extent than single doses. Absorption is believed to be mainly from the upper intestinal tract.

Allithiamine has been found to be more rapidly absorbed from the intestine than thiamine itself, and this gives higher blood levels of thiamine with greater rapidity. Experiments have been carried out with animals and man using dithiopropylthiamine, a compound with the same structure as allithiamine, but with the propyl replacing the allyl group (*Nutrition Reviews* **18,** *181* (*1960*)). Dithiopropylthiamine, by virtue of its rapid intestinal absorption, causes far more rapid attainment of high blood levels of thiamine and liver cocarboxylase than thiamine itself.

In the U.S.A. thiamine deficiency is by no means a rarity. It is confined mainly to the alcoholic population. Alcoholism is an increasingly prevalent condition and several clinical features previously believed to be due to alcoholic poisoning are now known to be due to nutritional deficiencies.

Wernicke's disease is characterized by eye signs (nystagmus, diplopia, paralysis of the externi recti muscles, and sometimes ophthalmoplegia), ataxia, and mental changes. Korsakoff's psychosis leads to a loss of memory of the immediate past and often to an elaborate confabulation which tends to conceal this amnesia. It is now generally agreed that any distinction between Wernicke's disease and Korsakoff's psychosis may be artificial in the alcoholic patient. Korsakoff's psychosis may be regarded as the psychotic component of Wernicke's disease (M. Victor and R. D. Adams, *Am. J. Clin. Nutrition* **9,** *379* (*1961*)). These authors report that in 62 out of 72 patients who presented with ocular palsy, ataxia, and confusion (and who survived for longer than a few days) the characteristic amnestic disorder of Korsakoff's psychosis became evident.

Similarly in patients with Korsakoff's psychosis in two state hospitals the stigmata of Wernicke's disease were found even years after their illness. Pathologically there is also an indication of the unity of the two diseases. If treated early, the signs

of the Wernicke-Korsakoff syndrome respond to thiamine alone even if alcohol is continued.

Of overriding importance in this syndrome is the fact that irreversible brain damage ensues rapidly, and therefore early recognition and treatment are vital. Prevention also calls for considerable public health ingenuity. Possibilities suggested have included fortification of alcoholic beverages with thiamine, frequent "immunization" of alcoholics with thiamine and development of a suitable depot carrier to reduce the frequency of these injections, and the provision by public health authorities of thiamine impregnated snacks on bar counters. The cost of any of these measures would almost certainly be less than the present very high cost of caring for those who have suffered from Wernicke-Korsakoff's disease.

Alcoholic polyneuropathy, similar to neuritic beriberi, is also a disease largely due to a nutritional thiamine deficiency.

Alcoholic amblyopia is similar to a condition seen in prisoner of war camps. In both, central scotomas are found and thiamine has been implicated as the deficiency.

The role of thiamine deficiency vis a vis deficiencies of pantothenic acid, riboflavin, vitamin B_6, and other vitamins in the "burning feet syndrome" has not been conclusively resolved (J. H. Walters, *Tr. Roy. Soc. Trop. Med. Hyg.* **60,** *128* (*1966*)). The spinal neuropathies reported from West Africa and in prisoners of war in the Far East may be due to deficiencies of B vitamins, but have not been proven to result from thiamine deficiency alone. In an outbreak of an ataxic neuropathy in an East African prison, Latham (*Brit. J. Nutrition* **18,** *129* (*1964*)) showed that the diet of the afflicted prisoners contained less than 0.4 mg. thiamine per 1,000 calories, but was also relatively deficient in certain other vitamins. It would not be surprising to find several deficiencies involved in a single neurological syndrome. The nervous system is after all a finely adjusted mechanism, utilizing a wide range of complex enzyme systems to control energy supplied to it. The prosthetic group of these enzymes is frequently a vitamin.

It could be predicted that in the years ahead more will be learned of the interrelationship between the vitamins. It is possible that certain syndromes will be found to be due to a particular "mix" of vitamin intakes in persons on an inadequate diet, and that particular staple foods favor the type of "mix" which leads to one or other of these syndromes. This might explain the clinical differences in certain geographic locales or among certain groups of persons. It is hoped that the great advances being made in unraveling the chemical properties and enzyme functions of vitamins like thiamine will not only clarify their physiological action but, allied with dietary investigations and clinical study in man, will be able to define more clearly the precise etiology of the various deficiency diseases and syndromes.

CHAPTER XV

PRESENT KNOWLEDGE OF RIBOFLAVIN

OLAF MICKELSEN, PH.D.

The *U. S. Department of Agriculture Household Food Consumption Survey of 1955* showed an average daily intake of 2.0 to 2.5 mg. riboflavin per person. This increase over 1936 was attributed to enriched cereals and greater consumption of milk and meat products. There was some relation between riboflavin intake and family income. Although the figures are well above the 1964 recommended allowances of the Food and Nutrition Board, they are subject to a number of limitations and should be interpreted with a certain amount of caution.

Riboflavin intake in many other countries of the world is frequently limited; so much so that ariboflavinosis is still a common nutritional deficiency. It is one of the more frequent in the Congo, and in many underdeveloped countries occurs among both military and civilian personnel.

"Shibi-gatchaki," a disease among a large percentage of the inhabitants of the northernmost province of the main island of Japan, has been reported due to a deficiency of riboflavin; the patients' condition improves with riboflavin supplements.

As a result of studies which revealed that many pregnant women from the lower socioeconomic strata of Jerusalem showed definite signs of ariboflavinosis, all flour milled in Israel after 1948 was fortified with (per kilogram) 2.5 mg. riboflavin, 2.5 g. calcium carbonate, and 30 g. heat-processed soymeal. This measure was effective. The improved condition of the pregnant women as evidenced by later surveys was attributed to the fact that 35 per cent of their riboflavin intake came from the enriched flour (K. Guggenheim, A. Brezezenski, J. Ilan, and B. Kallner, *Am. J. Clin. Nutrition* **7**, *526* (*1959*)).

Skin changes, especially at the mucosal-epidermal junction, still appear to be the primary clinical diagnostic criterion for ariboflavinosis among human subjects. Changes in blood levels of the vitamin provide only a suggestion as to the body's store of riboflavin.

A normochromic and normocytic anemia has been reported in patients fed a synthetic diet severely deficient in riboflavin (*Nutrition Reviews* **23**, *197* (*1965*)). The anemia and the deficiency were accentuated by galactoflavin, a riboflavin antagonist. The anemia was not improved by iron-dextran or pyridoxine, but promptly responded to riboflavin therapy.

It was suggested on the basis of only one assay for erythropoietin in one patient that riboflavin is a "cofactor for erythropoietin action." This anemia is not a regularly described component of the naturally occurring form of human riboflavin deficiency (V. P. Sydenstricker, *Am. J. Pub. Health* **31**, *344* (*1941*)).

Whether a riboflavin deficiency produces an anemia in animals is becoming more questionable. There were a number of early reports of anemia in riboflavin deficient rats, mice, dogs, foxes, and pigs. For some of these species, *e.g.* pigs, later work using rations containing folic acid and vitamin B_{12} resulted in a riboflavin deficiency with no hematological changes (S. W. Terrill, *J. Animal Sci.* **14**, *593* (*1955*)).

Baboons fed a diet free of riboflavin for two to four months had hemoglobin levels averaging 6.4 g. per 100 ml. The *Cebus* monkey differs in this respect from the baboon. Monkeys fed a ration very low in riboflavin showed no signs of anemia until at the point of death. This anemia was probably due to the accompanying anorexia. Riboflavin deficiency anemia in monkeys reported earlier may have been due to a folic acid deficiency (*Nutrition Reviews* **23**, 87 (*1965*)).

Circumstantial support for the suggestion that anemia attributed to a riboflavin deficiency may be due to another nutrient comes from the absence of anemia in cats severely deficient in riboflavin (S. N. Gershoff, S. B. Andrus, and D. M. Hegsted, *J. Nutrition* **68**, 75 (*1959*)). In that study, anorexia, body weight loss, cataracts, testicular hypoplasia, fatty livers, and mild skin changes were the primary symptoms.

No signs of anemia or abnormalities of other blood constituents were seen in guinea pigs maintained as long as 13 weeks on a diet free of riboflavin (H. Hara, *J. Vitaminol.* **6**, 24 (*1960*)). None of the deficient animals showed pronounced symptoms. The hearts were most affected—vacuolar degeneration of muscle cells with abnormal deposits of glycogen were seen frequently. Many heart muscle cells were atrophied and separated from each other by hemorrhages or edema.

A deficiency of riboflavin in the pregnant rat, when accentuated with injections of galactoflavin, resulted in the birth of young whose incisor teeth became so maloccluded that, for survival purposes, they had to be cut (F. M. Deuschle, E. Takacs, and J. Warkany, *J. Dent. Res.* **40**, 366 (*1961*)). Attempts to correlate these alterations with enzymatic changes during fetal development resulted in the suggestion "that a critically low level of FAD (flavin adenine dinucleotide) may be the cause of the embryo malformations . . ." (*see Nutrition Reviews* **21**, 24 (*1963*)). There may be some question as to whether the reduction in FAD is really the primary biochemical abnormality. This suggestion is based on the earlier observation that young rats fed a diet deficient in riboflavin showed a depletion of FMN (flavin mononucleotide) rather than FAD.

When pregnant mice were fed a riboflavin deficient ration containing galactoflavin (H. Kalter, *Pediatrics* **23**, 222 (*1959*)), the young showed a large number of abnormalities involving the skeleton, brain, and esophagus. The extent and severity varied with the strains of mice.

The requirement for riboflavin has been reviewed by F. Bro-Rasmussen (*Nutrition Abst. Rev.* **28**, 1, 367 (*1958*)). He points out that whenever dietary protein is adequate, a deficiency of riboflavin does not occur in adult human subjects with daily intakes above 0.5 to 0.8 mg. The riboflavin requirement is intimately related to caloric intake—for adults, 250 to 270 μg. per 1,000 calories.

His evidence appears to explain earlier reports of an increase in riboflavin requirement with an increase in dietary fat. These reports are based entirely on animal studies, and the explanation pertains only to animals such as dogs and poultry where, Bro-Rasmussen says, the intestinal flora has little effect on the riboflavin requirement. For other animals, *e.g.* the rat and cat, intestinal synthesis of the vitamin may be markedly influenced by the composition of the diet. This, in turn, may be mirrored in the animal's riboflavin requirement.

For growing organisms, the requirement for riboflavin (presumably to saturate the tissues) is approximately 700 μg. per 1,000 calories. This requirement is surprisingly uniform for species ranging from mice through calves and horses. The constancy of the association between caloric intake and riboflavin requirement led the Food and Nutrition Board of the National Academy of Sciences (*National Academy of Sciences –National Research Council publication 1146. Washington, D. C., 1964*) to revise the basis for its recommendations concerning this vitamin. The Board previously had linked the riboflavin requirement to the protein level of the diet. The 1964 publication states that "riboflavin allowances have been computed ... as 0.6 mg/1000 calories." This change, however, makes very little difference in the recommended allowances.

Little has been done to evaluate the riboflavin requirement of germfree animals. One group (T. D. Luckey, J. R. Pleasents, and J. A. Reyniers, *J. Nutrition* **55,** *105* (1955)) found that germfree chicks fed a ration without riboflavin grew as rapidly as conventional birds fed the same ration. Mortality set in earlier and was slightly greater among the germfree birds. There were, however, no differences in concentrations of a variety of vitamins in the livers and cecal contents of the two groups. These observations fit in with Bro-Rasmussen's claim that the chick's gastrointestinal flora plays only a minor role in meeting nutritional requirements.

Despite a very high intake, riboflavin concentration in the livers of germfree guinea pigs was reported to be half that of normal controls (Hara, *loc. cit.*).

Although the statement has been made that approximately twice as much dietary riboflavin is required for tissue saturation as for maximum growth (Bro-Rasmussen, *loc. cit.*), the factor may be as high as five. Carcasses of rats showed increasing riboflavin concentrations with daily intakes up to 100 μg. However, there was no essential difference in growth rates of male rats receiving daily intakes above 20 μg. (O. A. Bessey, O. H. Lowry, E. B. Davis, and J. L. Dorn, *J. Nutrition* **64,** *185* (1958)).

Besides dietary riboflavin, unknown factors appear to influence tissue concentration. For the same intakes, female rats showed lower body weight gains and higher carcass concentrations. Higher concentrations were secured when commercial rather than purified rations were used. Although female rats had slightly higher carcass concentrations of riboflavin for the same intakes, males had higher maximum concentrations in their livers.

Cold environmental temperatures appear to have little or only minimal influence on the riboflavin requirement of animals. Some reports dispute this conclusion. The different experimental conditions in each investigation make comparison of results almost impossible.

Study of the influence of genetic factors on riboflavin requirement has been extended to White Leghorn hens which were unable to incorporate an adequate amount of riboflavin in their eggs. The latter contained so little riboflavin that the embryos died by the fourteenth day of incubation. Injection of riboflavin into the eggs produced normal chicks. A recessive gene prevented transfer of adequate amounts of riboflavin from the ration to the egg. This was associated with a failure of riboflavin blood levels to increase in the hen at the onset of laying. Attempts to increase blood levels by intracardiac injection of the vitamin or subcutaneous injections of estrogens proved fruitless (J. W. Cowan, R. V. Boucher, and E. G. Buss, *Poultry Sci.* **40,** *1390* (1961); *Nutrition Reviews* **22,** *273* (1964)).

Urinary excretion of riboflavin by normal human subjects is related to intake. When these two variables are plotted, there is a sharp break in the curve at a daily intake of 1 to 1.5 mg. riboflavin. For children, the break occurs at an intake of 0.6 to 0.7 mg., for pregnant women, at 1.5 to 2.0 mg. (Bro-Rasmussen, *loc. cit.*). At intakes below that "critical" point, the slope of the excretion curve is almost parallel to the intake axis and not very far above it. With intakes above that level, the rate of excretion increases much more rapidly.

For normal subjects maintained over extended periods on the same vitamin intake, there is no evidence that riboflavin excretion is an individual characteristic.

Many studies have shown an increased excretion of riboflavin whenever the subject was in negative nitrogen balance, and it has been stated that "the flavoproteins may be a part of the labile rather than stable proteins" in the body (J. M. Smith *et al., J. Nutrition* **69,** *85* (*1959*)). Many situations can be explained on such a basis.

There is, however, some evidence that makes it difficult to accept a causal relationship between nitrogen loss from the body and riboflavin excretion. This is based on (1) the reduced urinary excretion of riboflavin which sets in on the third day when individuals receive no food but water ad libitum; (2) the great variability in the ratio of riboflavin-to-nitrogen excretion seen in subjects who presumably were in the same nutritional condition at the start of periods during which a negative nitrogen balance occurred (*e.g.* bed rest); and (3) the low riboflavin excretion when acute thiamine deficiency produces a marked loss of weight and presumably also a marked loss of nitrogen (R. G. Tucker, O. Mickelsen, and A. Keys, *J. Nutrition* **72,** *251* (*1960*)).

Hard physical work with an adequate caloric and a constant riboflavin intake reduced young men's urinary riboflavin excretion. The reduction was progressive, so that by the fourth day of hard work excretion was 25 per cent that of the control period. If the hard work was extended, riboflavin excretion started to increase, so that by the tenth day it was two-thirds the control value. The inhibitory effect of hard work appears to be carried over into periods of starvation. When hard physical work was combined with the absence of food, riboflavin excretion increased threefold; when these men were as inactive as possible (without any food), the increase was sevenfold.

Futher evidence for the absence of a constant relation between urinary riboflavin and nitrogen excretion comes from the observation that during the first day when no food is eaten, the increase in excretion does not occur until 13 to 20 hours after the last meal (H. G. Windmueller, A. A. Anderson, and Mickelsen, *Am. J. Clin. Nutrition* **15,** *73* (*1964*)). Toward the end of the fast (24

to 37 hours after the last meal), the excretion rate for riboflavin was ten to 15 times what it had been the day before the fast started.

Riboflavin excretion during periods of semi-starvation (food intake inadequate to maintain body weight) also shows a number of peculiarities that do not correlate with nitrogen excretion. When normal young men were semi-starved with a diet adequate in all respects except calories, the urinary riboflavin excretion was slightly lower than expected (A. Keys *et al., The Biology of Human Starvation, vol. 1, p. 473. University of Minnesota Press, Minneapolis, 1950*). Reduced excretion occurred despite the fact that body tissue was being metabolized, as evidenced by a negative nitrogen balance. On the assumption that catabolism of body tissue was occurring at a more or less uniform rate throughout the six months of semi-starvation, riboflavin accruing from the catabolized tissue should have been four times the observed urinary excretion. These results suggest that riboflavin excretion differs in acute and semi-starvation.

During rehabilitation from the preceding starvation, the subjects excreted more riboflavin in their urine than anticipated on the basis of their intake. This was true at both the sixth and twelfth weeks of rehabilitation. It was anticipated that urinary excretion would have been smaller than normal because of the extra riboflavin being stored in the regenerating tissue.

The nature of the diet appears to influence urinary excretion. When riboflavin intake was constant (630 to 622 μg. per day), excretion was much greater during the week that a diet high in meat was consumed than when a diet low in meat was fed (S. Iinuma, *J. Vitaminol.* **1,** *90* (*1955*)). During the week the diet with 14 per cent of calories from meat was eaten, urinary riboflavin was fairly constant at 159 μg. per 24 hours. The following week when the diet contained 58 per cent of calories from meat and eggs, excretion increased progressively from 250 to 500 μg. Stool riboflavin values were the same during both of these periods. However, when a vegetable diet was eaten, fecal riboflavin increased fivefold. The lack of correlation between stool and urinary excretion suggests that none of the riboflavin synthesized in the intestinal tract was contributing to urinary excretion.

There is evidence that more riboflavin is excreted in the urine of normal young men when they are fed a synthetic-type diet than when a regular diet with the same riboflavin content is fed (Tucker, Mickelsen, and Keys, *loc. cit.*).

Chapter XVI

PRESENT KNOWLEDGE OF VITAMIN B$_6$

M. A. Williams, Ph.D.

The chemistry, nutritional and metabolic effects, and enzymatic functions of vitamin B$_6$ have been very completely summarized (*Vitamins and Hormones* **22,** *361* (*1964*)) by the papers presented at the International Symposium on Vitamin B$_6$ in honor of Professor Paul György, who first identified vitamin B$_6$ as a separate member of the B-vitamin complex. A summary of recent research on the mechanisms of pyridoxal catalysis is presented in *Chemical and Biological Aspects of Pyridoxal Catalysis, E. E. Snell et al., Editors. Pergamon Press, New York, 1963,* as well as the recent review by P. Fasella (*Ann. Rev. Biochem.* **36,** *185* (*1967*)). The biochemical and physiological effects of B$_6$ deficiency in man and criteria for evaluation of and physiological effects of vitamin B$_6$ nutrition have been discussed by H. Linkswiler (*Am. J. Clin. Nutrition* **20,** *547* (*1967*)). P. Holtz and D. Palm have also made an extensive review of physiological effects of vitamin B$_6$ in relation to its enzymatic functions (*Pharmacol. Rev.* **16,** *113* (*1964*)). Methods for determination of B$_6$ and its coenzyme forms have been reviewed by C. A. Storvick, E. M. Benson, M. A. Edwards, and M. J. Woodring in *Methods of Biochemical Analysis* **12,** *183* (*1964*).

With respect to its enzymatic functions, it is valid to say that the vitamin, as pyridoxal phosphate (PLP) or pyridoxamine phosphate (PMP), is involved in synthesis and/or catabolism of all amino acids. In higher animals, this includes (1) synthesis of all non-essential amino acids and transamination of the keto-analogues of essential amino acids; (2) decarboxylation of many amino acids; (3) interconversion of glycine and serine, which relates to pro-duction of 1-C units for methyl group synthesis; (4) formation of cysteine from methionine, and its conversion to taurine; (5) synthesis of dihydrosphingosine, the precursor of sphingosine; and (6) synthesis of delta-aminolevulinic acid (ALA), from which cellular porphyrin compounds, including hemoglobin, myoglobin, and the cytochromes, are formed. A recently investigated reaction, the mechanism not fully established, is coupled oxidative deamination and decarboxylation of glycine, which occurs in chicken liver as in microorganisms. In this reaction, glycine is converted to carbon dioxide, ammonia, and hydroxymethyl-tetrahydrofolic acid.

In addition, pyridoxal phosphate is an essential part of the enzyme glycogen phosphorylase, although its specific function has not yet been clarified.

Glycine. The importance of vitamin B$_6$ in metabolism of glycine and serine was emphasized by the observation that B$_6$ deficiency caused oxaluria in cats and rats, with development of renal oxalate calculi (S. N. Gershoff and F. F. Faragalla, *J. Biol. Chem.* **234,** *239* (*1959*)). The increased excretion of oxalate may reflect decreased ability to form glycine from glyoxylate or from glycolate. A decrease in the activity of the transaminase catalyzing glycine synthesis from glyoxylate and alanine or glutamate has been reported in rats deficient in B$_6$ (J. S. Thompson and K. E. Richardson, *Arch. Biochem. Biophys.* **117,** *599* (*1966*)). Supplementation with additional pyridoxine decreased oxalate excretion in human beings with a tendency to form renal oxalate stones, although these subjects had been receiving adequate B$_6$ and were excreting only normal amounts of oxalate (Gershoff and E. L. Prien, *Am. J. Clin. Nutrition* **8,** *812 (1960)*).

These results suggest the possibility that relatively low B$_6$ intakes may be a factor in the greater incidence of vesical oxalate calculi in children in parts of the world where poor nutrition is prevalent. This condition is not to be confused with the human genetic disorder, primary hyperoxaluria.

Sulfur amino acids. The discovery of the central role of vitamin B$_6$ in amino acid metabolism explained why diets high in protein, especially methionine, increase the requirement for the vitamin. However, the increased requirement implies that high amino acid intakes produce either an increased loss of the vitamin from the cell or increased levels of PLP-enzymes, and thus a greater requirement for PLP. There is little evidence for the first possibility, which can be established definitely only by studies with isotopically labeled B$_6$. It has been clearly demonstrated, however, that high protein intakes produce adaptive increases in activity levels of PLP-enzymes in amino acid catabolism (J. E. Wergedal and A. E. Harper, *J. Biol. Chem.* **239,** *1956 (1964)*).

Activity of several of the PLP-enzymes which function in the metabolism of methionine and cysteine is especially sensitive to changes in sulfur amino acid intake. Dietary cystine can replace a major portion of higher animals' dietary requirement for methionine. Only recently has an enzymatic basis for this regulation been proposed. Conversion of methionine to cysteine involves formation of cystathionine from homocysteine and serine, a reaction catalyzed by the PLP-enzyme, cystathionine synthase. Cystathionine, in turn, is split to yield cysteine, with a transfer of homocysteine sulfur to the carbon chain of the serine portion of cystathionine. This reaction is catalyzed by the PLP-enzyme, cystathionase.

Injections of methionine or feeding diets high in methionine for a short period produced a 50 per cent increase in activity of liver cystathionase in rats (O. Trautmann and F. Chatagner, *Bull. Soc. Chim. Biol.* **46,** *129 (1964)*). The increased activity resulted, at least in part, from an increase in the amount of enzyme protein. Recently, A. Kato and co-workers (*J. Biochem.* **59,** *34, 40 (1966)*) reported that a metabolite of cystine inhibited *in vitro* the activity of cystathionine synthase.

J. Finkelstein and S. H. Mudd (*J. Biol. Chem.* **242,** *873 (1967)*) observed that the liver content of cystathionine synthase was reduced by feeding cystine and was increased by feeding or injection of methionine. Injection of various levels of methionine produced corresponding increases in activity of cystathionine synthase, as well as cystathionase and methionine activating enzyme. Methionine activating enzyme catalyzes formation of S-adenosylmethionine from methionine. Feeding cystine also decreased activity of cystathionase and methionine activating enzyme, but these decreases were less than the decrease in synthase activity.

Finkelstein and Mudd suggested that metabolic regulation of sulfur amino acids may be based on the activity of cystathionine synthase.

Homocystinuria, a genetic defect in human beings resulting in mental retardation, is characterized by abnormal urinary excretion of homocystine. In cases studied thus far, there was a large decrease in activity of liver cystathionine synthase. The concentration of brain cystathionine was also lower in these patients, and this may be a factor in mental retardation. Cystathionine has been suggested as a post-synaptic inhibitory agent (R. Werman, R. A. Davidoff, and M. H. Aprison, *Life Sci.* **5,** *1431 (1966)*).

The decrease in cystathionine synthase activity produced by feeding cystine is a potential complication in treating patients with homocystinuria. This treatment would be expected to reduce even more the synthase activity, already abnormally low. An additional decrease might intensify any changes resulting from a deficiency of tissue cystathionine, since cystathionine may have other functions than as a cysteine precursor.

Cystathioninuria, another human metabolic defect in sulfur amino acid metabolism, results in an increase in urinary cystathionine (G. W. Frimpter, A. J. Greenberg, M. Hilgartner, and F. Fuchs, *Am. J. Dis. Child.* **113**, *115* (*1967*)). This condition is characterized by a defect in the enzyme cystathionase. High doses of pyridoxine (orally or intramuscularly) reduced concentration of cystathionine in blood and urine of three patients. Comparison of conversion of cystathionine to cysteine by liver homogenates from biopsy specimens showed that it was much less in homogenates from these patients than in normal controls.

Addition of excess PLP to the assay did not increase conversion by normal tissue, but did in homogenates from these patients, although cysteine formation was still subnormal. The subjects showed no clinical signs of B_6 deficiency, and metabolism of a tryptophan load was normal. The results were interpreted to indicate that a structural alteration in the apoenzyme had resulted in weaker binding of PLP, so that an increase in PLP concentration would increase the amount of enzyme-coenzyme complex. Changes in the structure of other PLP-enzymes with a decrease in binding of PLP could be responsible for other B_6 dependency syndromes which require large amounts of pyridoxine for correction.

Antibody and protein synthesis. Antibody formation is reduced in B_6 deficiency, and this can be related to the fact that the deficiency inhibits incorporation of amino acids into protein, both *in vivo* and *in vitro*. The reduced incorporation is accompanied by a decrease in tissue polysomes and reduced incorporation of orotic acid into ribosomal RNA (M. Montjar, A. E. Axelrod, and A. C. Trakatellis, *J. Nutrition* **85**, *45* (*1965*)). Furthermore, B_6 deficiency af-

fects incorporation of various nucleic acid precursors into DNA in rats, and thus results in a decrease in spleen DNA concentration.

Consequently, B_6 deficiency appears to lower antibody production by reducing synthesis of nucleic acids required for cells which form antibodies, as well as reducing synthesis of immune proteins. The decreased absorption of vitamin B_{12} in rats deficient in B_6 may also be a factor altering nucleic acid synthesis (J. M. Hsu and B. F. Chow, *Arch. Biochem. Biophys.* **72**, *322* (*1957*)).

Aminolevulinic acid synthesis. Involvement of PLP in synthesis of delta-aminolevulinic acid (ALA) explains the anemia observed in animals deficient in pyridoxine. ALA, precursor of heme and other porphyrin compounds, is formed by condensation of succinyl CoA and glycine. The enzyme catalyzing this reaction, ALA-synthetase, is a PLP-enzyme. Synthesis of ALA is reduced in red blood cells of ducklings deficient in pyridoxine.

Adding PLP to these cells increased synthesis of heme from glycine and succinate (D. A. Richert and M. P. Schulman, *Am. J. Clin. Nutrition* **7**, *416* (*1959*)). It is not yet known whether limited formation of ALA is a factor in the type of human anemia which responds to large doses of pyridoxine. One patient with this type of anemia, however, used more ALA than glycine for porphyrin synthesis (J. W. Harris and D. L. Horrigan, *Vitamins and Hormones* **22**, *721* (*1964*)). Such anemias may represent a genetic metabolic error which increases dependency of erythropoiesis on B_6, perhaps through ALA synthesis.

Sphingosine. PLP was reported to stimulate synthesis of dihydrosphingosine in rat brain extracts (R. O. Brady, J. V. Formica, and G. J. Korval, *J. Biol. Chem.* **233**, *26*, *1072* (*1958*)). Dihydrosphingosine, precursor of the phospholipid base sphingosine, appeared to be formed from addition of palmitaldehyde to the C-2 of serine; the carboxyl group of serine is lost as carbon dioxide. P. E. Braun and E. E. Snell (*Proc. Nat. Acad. Sci.* **58,** *298* (*1967*)) have investigated this reaction in more detail in the yeast, *Hansenula ciferri,* and found that dihydrosphingosine was formed by condensation of palmityl CoA and serine. Treatment of the active enzyme extract with cysteine reduced activity by 80 per cent, and PLP restored it. Condensation of palmityl CoA and serine is analogous to the formation of delta-aminolevulinic acid from succinyl CoA and glycine.

Phosphorylase. The finding that PLP was an essential part of glycogen phosphorylase suggested new functions for this coenzyme, which up to this time was associated chiefly with enzymes of amino acid metabolism. T. Baranowski, B. Illingworth, D. H. Brown, and C. F. Cori (*Biochim. Biophys. Acta* **25,** *16* (*1957*)) found that PLP was present in rabbit muscle phosphorylase. Cori and Illingworth (*Proc. Nat. Acad. Sci.* **43,** *547* (*1957*)) showed that PLP was required for catalytic activity.

Vitamin B$_6$ deficiency decreased levels of skeletal muscle phosphorylase in the rat and mouse, but adding PLP to muscle preparations did not increase enzyme activity. This suggested that synthesis of the apoenzyme is reduced in deficient animals.

Liver and adrenal phosphorylase also decreased. Muscle glycogen levels were normal or slightly reduced in deficient rats. This is in contrast to the higher levels of muscle glycogen in type V glycogen storage disease in human beings, when muscle phosphorylase is absent.

A major part of muscle vitamin B$_6$ may be present as PLP bound to phosphorylase, since B$_6$ deficiency causes approximately a 35 per cent decrease in both muscle phosphorylase activity and B$_6$ content. In other tissues, phosphorylase activity is much lower, but B$_6$ content is higher. Consequently, the proportion of B$_6$ bound to phosphorylase must be much lower in these tissues, whereas a major part of muscle B$_6$ would occur in phosphorylase.

Phosphorylase shows none of the characteristic enzymatic functions of PLP dependent enzymes. E. H. Fischer and E. G. Krebs (*Fed. Proc.* **25,** *1511* (*1966*)) have proposed the following alternatives for the action of PLP in phosphorylase: (a) PLP acts in the control of enzyme activity, although not directly concerned in catalysis; (b) PLP is a structural part of the protein and may contribute to its stability or serve as a storage form of B$_6$; (c) PLP is directly involved in catalysis, not through the aldehyde or phenolic groups, but possibly through the ring nitrogen.

Metabolism of vitamin B$_6$. Availability of radioactively labeled forms of B$_6$ will make possible more detailed and quantitative studies on its metabolism. Experiments with pyridoxine labeled with tritium have recently been published. A. M. Huber and Gershoff (*J. Nutrition* **87,** *407* (*1966*)) found that the pituitary showed the highest uptake of pyridoxine per gram of tissue as well as the most rapid loss when the rats were transferred to a pyridoxine deficient diet. This indicates that pituitary metabolism may be greatly changed in pyridoxine deficiency.

D. A. Vaughan and R. L. Winders (*Metabolism* **15,** *676* (*1966*)) reported that deoxypyridoxine appeared to block *in vivo* some of the sites available for attachment of ^{3}H-pyridoxine, since tritium excretion was greater in rats fed a deficient diet plus deoxypyridoxine than in those fed the deficient diet without the antagonist. S. Johansson, S. Lindstedt, and U. Register (*Am. J. Physiol.* **210,** *1086* (*1966*)) reported that urinary excretion of tritium the first day after injection of tritiated pyridoxine increased as dietary pyridoxine intake increased, but the elimination rate after the first day was not significantly changed by the level of pyridoxine fed.

Lipid metabolism. A role for pyridoxine in fatty acid or essential fatty acid metabolism is still unclear, although PLP is indirectly involved in fatty acid metabolism via synthesis of sphingosine, serine, ethanolamine, and choline. The original suggestion that essential fatty acid metabolism might be altered in B_6 deficiency was based on a superficial resemblance between skin lesions of essential fatty acid deficiency and pyridoxine deficiency. Yet, histologically, the two conditions are very different, and feeding arachidonate does not cure the lesions of B_6 deficiency. (V. Ramalingaswami and H. M. Sinclair, *J. Invest. Dermat.* **20,** *81 (1953)*).

Some evidence for a direct effect of B_6 in fat metabolism was provided by the observation that PLP stimulated incorporation of ^{14}C-acetate into fatty acids by mitochondrial extracts from beef liver. The response of these extracts to PLP varied, however. In contrast, addition of PLP depressed acetate incorporation into fatty acids by intact mitochondria (W. Stoffel, *Hoppe Seyler's Z. f. Physiol. Chem.* **333,** *71 (1963)*).

Recently, A. Goswami and J. C. Coniglio (*Proceedings of the Seventh International Congress of Nutrition, Hamburg, p. 253, 1966*) found that PLP stimulated incorporation of ^{14}C-acetyl CoA into arachidonate and docosahexaenoate by liver microsomes, as well as into long chain fatty acids in both microsomes and mitochondria. This is the most direct evidence for a function of PLP in fatty acid synthesis.

Dental caries. Hamsters and monkeys fed diets deficient in B_6 show an increase in dental caries. Evidence for an effect of B_6 on dental caries in man is still not definite, although limited clinical studies indicate that pyridoxine supplementation may have a protective effect (R. W. Hillman, *Vitamins and Hormones* **22,** *695 (1964)*).

Vitamin B_6 nutrition in human beings. The minimum requirement for young men has been established at 1.25 mg. per day (30 g. protein per day) or 1.50 mg. per day (100 g. protein per day) with either a purified formula diet supplying 0.06 mg. of B_6, unless supplemented, or with a diet of natural foods (H. E. Sauberlich, *Vitamins and Hormones* **22,** *807 (1964)*). With these levels of pyridoxine, normal levels of xanthurenic acid were excreted after a tryptophan load test.

Recommended intakes were about 1.5 mg. per day for low protein diets and 1.75 to 2.0 mg. per day for high protein diets. With the unsupplemented formula diet described above, abnormal xanthurenic acid excretion occurred within one week with the 100 g. diet and after six weeks with the 30 g. protein diet. Encephalographic abnormalities appeared after 21 days with either the high or low protein diets. These changes disappeared with pyridoxine treatment, but the speed of recovery was not a direct function of the amount or duration of treatment.

N. Yess *et al.* (*J. Nutrition* **84,** *229 (1964)*) found abnormal xanthurenic acid excretion in young men after two to 15 days of feeding a diet providing 100 g. protein and 0.16 mg. B_6 per day. Kynurenine and HO-kynurenine were also excreted in larger amounts, with HO-kynurenine the largest as the deficiency progressed.

Various tests for biochemical evaluation of vitamin B_6 nutrition continue to receive much needed attention. Excretion of xanthurenic acid after a load of tryptophan is still one of the most widely used, although comparison of results of different experiments is often difficult because of differences in analytical techniques and in the amount and form (DL- or L-) of tryptophan given. A standard dose of 2 g. L-tryptophan has been recommended for studies with adults, with a recommendation of 50 mg. per kilogram for infants.

An important criticism of the tryptophan load test, especially with larger amounts, is the possibility (a) that tryptophan may bind tissue PLP, *i.e.*, the test itself may produce a temporary deficiency of PLP for enzymatic functions (P. A. M. Hughes and D. N. Raine, *Clin. Chim. Acta* **14,** *399 (1966)*) or (b) that higher doses of tryptophan may increase the level of tryptophan pyrrolase relative to levels of other enzymes in kynurenine metabolism. This consequently would produce an increase in excretion of kynurenine and other metabolites, even in subjects with adequate vitamin B$_6$ intakes. A 2 g. load of L-tryptophan does not affect the level of tryptophan pyrrolase (K. Altman and O. Greengard, *J. Clin. Invest.* **45,** *1527* (*1966*)). Liver tryptophan pyrrolase may be elevated, however, in conditions which increase adrenal glucocorticoid secretion.

The basis for the excretion of xanthurenic acid as an index of vitamin B$_6$ deficiency depends upon the reactions involved in conversion of tryptophan to niacin, which are as follows:

$$\text{tryptophan} \xrightarrow{(1)} \text{kynurenine} \xrightarrow{(2)}$$

$$\text{3-HO-kynurenine} \xrightarrow{(3)}$$

$$\text{3-HO-anthranilic acid} \xrightarrow{(4)} \text{niacin.}$$

Kynureninase, the enzyme which catalyzes reaction 3, is a PLP-enzyme. Vitamin B$_6$ deficiency reduces the level of kynureninase activity so that more kynurenine and HO-kynurenine would be available for metabolism by other pathways, such as conversion to xanthurenic acid. Formation of xanthurenic acid, however, also involves a PLP dependent enzyme, kynurenine transaminase. One would expect that xanthurenic acid excretion would also be reduced in B$_6$ deficiency.

A possible explanation for a greater xanthurenic acid excretion was provided by N. Ogasawara, Y. Hagino, and Y. Kotake (*J. Biochem.* **52,** *162* (*1962*)). They found that kynureninase activity, which was principally in the "soluble" fraction of the cell, decreased by 75 per cent in rats deficient in pyridoxine, but kynurenine transaminase activity, which was chiefly mitochondrial, decreased by only 50 per cent. The depression in transaminase activity reflected chiefly a decrease in PLP, not in apoenzyme.

Another test of B$_6$ nutritional status is the effect of vitamin B$_6$ depletion and repletion on activity of glutamic-oxaloacetic (GOT) and glutamic-pyruvic (GPT) transaminases in different blood components. In most instances, the transaminase activity decreased during the deficiency, but the rate of increase during repletion varied with differences in degree of deficiency, amount of pyridoxine supplementation, and composition of the basal diet. GOT activity in erythrocytes appeared the most sensitive to depletion or repletion.

A significant decrease occurred in young men after only four days of deficiency with a diet supplying 150 g. protein per day. At this time, only small changes appeared in tryptophan metabolism (H. Linkswiler, *Am. J. Clin. Nutrition* **20,** *547* (*1967*)). In rats, GOT activity in whole blood hemolyzates appeared to be a better measure of B$_6$ intake than liver transaminase and responded linearly (log scale) to graded intakes of pyridoxine (M. C. Cheney and G. H. Beaton, *Canad. J. Physiol. Pharmacol.* **43,** *591* (*1965*)). However, blood GPT appeared more sensitive to B$_6$ deprivation.

Excretion of 4-pyridoxic acid, a major metabolite of vitamin B$_6$, is also used as an index of B$_6$ intake, since it decreases rapidly during depletion and increases with repletion. Blood levels of vitamin B$_6$ and its coenzyme forms reflect B$_6$ intake, but methodological difficulties in extraction, when blood is the test material, have limited the usefulness of this test.

Determination of vitamin B$_6$ in food. In the determination of B$_6$ in foods, the greatest improvement has been development of column chromatographic procedures by Dowex ion-exchange for separation of its different components. The column eluates are then analyzed by procedures suited to the vitamin form present in the eluate. Microbiological assay is still the principal method, although methods based on the fluorescence of pyridoxal cyanohydrin also have great sensitivity. The potential diffi-

culty with fluorescence procedures, however, is interference by other fluorescent
material in the eluates. In addition, as in
all analyses, complete extraction of the substance is a major problem. In determining
B_6 components, the problem is even greater
because of the variety of forms in which the
vitamin may occur.

Determination of the total B_6 content
from a summation of the separated components appears to give more reliable values
than a determination on the unchromato-
graphed extract, especially with products
high in starch, since chromatography re-
moves products of starch hydrolysis that
stimulate yeast growth. This chromatographic method of E. W. Toepfer and co-
workers was developed initially for food
products, especially plants. V. F. Thiele
and M. Brin (*J. Nutrition* **90**, *347* (*1966*))
have modified this procedure for use with
animal tissues.

Chapter XVII

PRESENT KNOWLEDGE OF HUMAN REQUIREMENTS FOR VITAMIN B$_{12}$

William J. Darby, M.D., Ph.D.

Prior to the identification of vitamin B$_{12}$ as the extrinsic factor, the minimal daily quantity of parenterally administered preparations which produced a maximal therapeutic response in patients with pernicious anemia defined a "unit." The only reliable assay procedure made use of the human with pernicious anemia. Hence, when crystalline vitamin B$_{12}$ initially was available, it was but logical for the late Randolph West and his collaborators to estimate the amount of the crystalline material which would be equivalent to this "unit."

From their early experience they (West and E. H. Reisner, Jr., *Am. J. Med.* **6,** *643* (*1949*)) estimated that 1 μg. of vitamin B$_{12}$ a day intramuscularly was a minimal effective dose. Subsequent investigations have revealed that this approximation is of an appropriate order, and the wealth of clinical experience based on the employment of parenteral dosages of approximately this level must be given proper weight in establishing the requirements for this vitamin.

A simple nutritional concept of pernicious anemia which seems valid is that of essentially an uncomplicated deficiency of vitamin B$_{12}$ conditioned by the lack of intrinsic factor and, hence, the inability to absorb the vitamin from ingested food. This validation rests on several types of evidence, of which particularly convincing is the comparison of the clinical development of B$_{12}$ deficiency in vegans, in patients following total gastrectomy (resulting in removal of intrinsic factor and interference with absorption of the vitamin) and the relapse following withholding of therapy from previously adequately treated patients with pernicious anemia. Simple experimental dietary deficiency of vitamin B$_{12}$ has not yet been produced in the adult human being under conditions of careful continuous observation. That such would be possible and could safely be undertaken is indicated by a comparison of observations on vegans, postgastrectomy subjects, and patients relapsing with pernicious anemia (W. J. Darby *et al.*, *Am. J. Clin. Nutrition* **6,** *513* (*1958*)).

Long adherence to a strictly vegetable dietary may result in a syndrome of glossitis, anemia, neurologic changes, and low serum levels of vitamin B$_{12}$, which responds to administration of this nutrient (F. Wokes, J. Badenoch, and H. M. Sinclair, *Am. J. Clin. Nutrition* **3,** *375* (*1955*); Wokes, *Proc. Nutrition Soc.* **15,** *134* (*1956*)). The onset of the similar syndrome of macrocytic anemia following total gastrectomy can be rather accurately timed. M. Paulson and J. C. Harvey (*J. Am. Med. Assn.* **156,** *1556* (*1954*)), for example, studied 27 patients who slowly developed macrocytosis (six months to seven years), anemia (one to eight years), and megaloblastic marrow (two to seven years) successively. Previously well treated patients with pernicious anemia who were regularly observed following interdiction of therapy required from four to 75 months to relapse hematologically. This is a time span almost exactly comparable to that required by gastrectomized patients or vegans to develop signs of B$_{12}$ deficiency.

It is of interest that the first hematologic evidence of relapse was macrocytosis, this occurring even before the appearance of well identified anemia. Hemopoiesis was impaired prior to the onset of the mildest evidences of glossitis or neurologic disturbance. From these and other data it appears valid to reason that the requirements of parenterally administered (or absorbed) vitamin B_{12} by the patient with pernicious anemia or gastrectomy should be similar to the requirements of the normal subject.

It has been of interest, therefore, to validate further the initial quantitative estimate made by West. Using long-adopted standards of initial response for adequately treated subjects it was found that parenterally administered doses less than 0.5 μg. per day of vitamin B_{12} produced in no instance an optimal rate of erythropoiesis; a dosage level of 0.5 μg. per day produced the expected erythropoiesis in two of five subjects; larger dosages up to 1.0 μg. produced maximal responses in four of six patients treated (Darby et al., Am. J. Med. **25,** 726 (1958)).

Maintenance studies in which relapsed patients were treated with 0.2 to 4.0 μg. daily parenterally of vitamin B_{12} for periods of three to 96 months and hemtaologic parameters (packed cell volume, hemoglobin, erythrocyte count, and MCV) assessed, led to the conclusion that from 0.5 to 2.0 μg. of vitamin B_{12} constituted the daily quantity of injected vitamin utilized for maintenance of maximal erythropoiesis (including disappearance of macrocytosis). The narrower range of 0.5 to 1.0 μg. sufficed for most subjects. Assuming these small doses of parenterally administered vitamin to be maximally utilized and accepting the existing evidence concerning efficiency of absorption of B_{12} by normal healthy individuals (G. B. J. Glass, Rev. Hematol. **10,** 137 (1955)) it was calculated that the minimal daily dietary need was 0.6 to 2.8 μg., with the range of 0.6 to 1.2 μg. sufficing for the majority.

The reasonableness of these estimates was supported by information obtained concerning the vitamin B_{12} content of dietaries of commonly used foodstuffs designed to meet the Recommended Dietary Allowances. High cost adequate, low cost adequate, and poor dietaries patterned after restricted diets consumed by a group of clinic patients were prepared and analyzed. These contained an average of 31.6, 16 and 2.7 μg. of vitamin B_{12} respectively (A. S. Mangay Chung et al., Am. J. Clin. Nutrition **9,** 573 (1961)).

Numerous measurements of the biological half life of vitamin B_{12} have been reported. Despite certain differences in interpretation all indicate a relatively long half life for the vitamin. Data of R. C. Bozian and co-workers (Bozian et al., Am. J. Clin. Nutrition **12,** 117 (1963)) revealed no significant difference in half life of vitamin B_{12} between normal subjects and patients with pernicious anemia. After two months or so the decay rate of radioactivity in the body was relatively constant. The biological half life corresponded to some 462 to 770 days, with a decay constant of 0.09 to 0.15 per cent of residual counts daily for healthy subjects, and from 0.11 to 0.17 per cent per day for patients with pernicious anemia.

Regardless of reported differences in the exact dimension of this constant, its existence indicates that the size of the residual body store of vitamin B_{12} is the major determinant of the quantity lost daily. Low levels of intake and small pool size are associated with excretion of small amounts of the factor. High levels of body stores result in excretion of larger quantities. It may be calculated that if initial body stores total some 4,000 μg. they would be depleted to a level of about 500 μg. (that estimated to be consistent with development of anemia) in about five years, assuming the daily decay rate of 0.1 per cent. Such is consistent with the clinical observations in relapse. Expressed in another way, to maintain a total body content of 5,000 μg. would require replacement of a loss of 5 μg. daily.

In order to ascertain whether such a quantity of vitamin B_{12} reasonably could be obtained from foodstuffs, R. M. Heyssel, Bozian, Darby, and M. C. Bell (Am. J.

Clin. Nutrition **18,** *176* (*1966*)) prepared meat of which the vitamin B_{12} was tagged with radioactive cobalt by feeding labeled cobalt chloride to lambs and subsequently slaughtering and butchering the animals. It was demonstrated that some 95 per cent of the radioactivity in the tissues fed corresponded to cyanocobalamine.

When meat was fed to normal subjects in an amount containing approximately 1 to 5 μg. of vitamin B_{12} absorption was similar to that observed when crystalline vitamin B_{12} was fed in like amounts. The data revealed that a block to absorption occurred at about 2.5 to 3 μg. per meal. Observations on absorption at successive meals indicated that there was no long-lasting saturation of B_{12} binding sites in the intestine nor residual interference with transport as a result of a prior meal. Hence, normal subjects readily could absorb an amount in excess of 6 μg. or so daily, if the three daily meals contained 3 to 5 μg. each.

Considerations outlined make it possible to approximate two defined levels of dietary standards: (1) Minimal dietary requirements as a floor on vitamin B_{12} needs sufficient to maintain health and normal hemopoiesis in most subjects with a small body pool of the vitamin. Using the absorption data from their observations on meat, Heyssel *et al.* (*loc. cit.*) are of the opinion that 0.9 to 1.8 μg. in food should provide a sufficient amount of the vitamin for the majority of individuals. (2) An intake to maintain high body stores at a level of 2 to 5 mg. for which the daily dietary intake would need to approximate 3 to 6 μg. or more.

Data on whole body counter measurements and their interpretation differ for different laboratories. However, workers differ more widely in their recognition of the variation in physiologic levels of nutriture than do the data on body loss. For example, H. C. Heinrich (*Seminars in Hematology* **1,** *199* (*1964*)) states that a human being must absorb at least 2.55 μg. of vitamin B_{12}

daily from a supply of 4 to 5 μg. or the clinical symptoms of vitamin B_{12} deficiency soon will develop. At the other extreme, L. W. Sullivan and V. Herbert (*New Engl. J. Med.* **272,** *340* (*1965*)) reported 0.1 μg. as the minimal daily requirement for vitamin B_{12}. The former high estimates failed to recognize the dependence of obligatory loss upon the total size of body stores of B_{12}. The latter gross underestimate of minimum requirement is based on observations in which the patients treated with 0.1 μg. exhibited neither maximal reticulocytosis nor even loss of morphologic evidence of B_{12} deficiency.

Unfortunately, the gradual evolution of biochemical knowledge is such that these long, tedious studies were initiated before it was possible to obtain reliable measures of vitamin B_{12} in blood and urine or of methylmalonate and other now recognized useful indices of nutrient level or metabolic function. In extending and refining studies of requirements it is essential properly to relate biochemical and morphologic findings to long term clinical observations.

All of the above data are limited to adults. There is no good evidence as to how estimates of requirements should vary during pregnancy. In view of the frequency with which folic acid responsive anemias are encountered in pregnancy and the infrequent occurrence of B_{12} responsive anemia, one might surmise that pregnancy does not greatly enhance B_{12} needs.

Similarly, there is little evidence concerning the vitamin B_{12} needs for growth. Earlier reports indicating enhancement of growth in children by administration of vitamin B_{12} have not been corroborated by more recent investigations. Finally, the physiologic significance of biochemically detectable metabolic variations (such as excretion of methylmalonate) in seemingly healthy, non-anemic individuals remains to be defined.

Chapter XVIII

PRESENT KNOWLEDGE OF ASCORBIC ACID (VITAMIN C)

C. G. King, Ph.D.

Vitamin C apparently was the first individual nutrient to be widely associated with disease. Primitive groups in many sections of the world knew of the requirement for fresh foods, particularly from plant sources, to prevent and cure the disease now recognized as scurvy. American Indians, for example, coveted fresh root tips and extracts of evergreen leaves in winter seasons and onion-like bulbs and leaves in early spring to prevent the symptoms characteristic of the vitamin deficiency. Research during the past 35 years, however, has developed most of the detailed knowledge of the vitamin as a single nutrient. Identification as a pure crystalline substance, methods of chemical analysis, and commercial synthesis from D-glucose were developments of the early 1930s (C. G. King, *Physiol. Rev.* **16,** *238* (*1936*); *Ann. N. Y. Acad. Sci.* **92,** Art. 1: *Vitamin C* (*1961*)).

The vitamin appears to be present and essential to the normal functioning of all cellular units in the higher plants and animals studied thus far, including subcellular structures such as ribosomes and mitochondria. The degree to which different tissues synthesize and distribute the substance to other tissues in the same organism has received very little attention in either plants or animals. In plants, however, it appears to play an essential role in photosynthesis and is formed rapidly in all of the most active cells during the initial germination stages in seeds. Several of the simpler sugars can be converted to ascorbic acid in plants, but in animals, D-glucose (chiefly) and D-galactose are the recognized precursors.

Among all animals studied thus far, only man and other primates, guinea pigs, the red vented bulbul bird and the fruit eating bat (both native to India) are dependent on food sources for the vitamin (R. N. Roy and B. C. Guha, *Nature* **182,** *319, 1689* (*1958*)). They are genetically deficient in the enzyme L-gulonolactone oxidase. Other animals synthesize ascorbic acid from glucose, via glucuronic acid and gulonic acid lactone (*Nutrition Reviews* **15,** *160* (*1957*)) and keep it under physiologic control if all essential nutrients are supplied.

The normal concentration of ascorbic acid in various tissues and body fluids of all the higher animals tends to follow a similar pattern but there are many moderate differences. Human milk, for example, generally contains three to four times as much vitamin C as found in cows' milk, unless the mother's diet is markedly deficient for a long period.

The tissue distribution and patterns of change during a deficient dietary intake are similar, so far as studied, in man and all the animals dependent upon a dietary intake. Muscle tissue is relatively low in ascorbic acid content, compared with glandular tissues. During depletion blood and urinary concentrations fall more rapidly and in greater degree—approaching zero—compared with blood cells and fixed tissues. The pituitary, adrenal cortex, corpus luteum, embryonic tissue, leucocytes, and glandular cells of the intestinal tract are particularly high and vary with the degree of activity. Pancreas, kidney, liver, thymus, salivary, spleen, and brain tissue are intermediate.

The rate of synthesis and excretion in rats can be greatly retarded or accelerated, depending upon the intake of other nutrients and special chemicals. Inanition or deficient intakes of thiamine or vitamin A cause a marked decrease in urinary excretion, milk alone induces a low level of excretion compared with a mixed diet containing essential oils such as carvone, and nearly all nerve depressants such as chloretone and barbiturates cause very large increases in synthesis and excretion. Certain hydrocarbons such as 3,4-benzpyrine are more active. Use of these techniques has greatly facilitated research on the synthesis and metabolism of the vitamin (C. G. King, R. R. Becker, H. H. Burns et al., see Nutrition Reviews 12, 155 (1954); 19, 48 (1961)).

The characteristic features of vitamin C deficiency, approximately in order of evidence, are: decreased urinary excretion, decreased plasma concentration, decreased tissue and leucocyte concentration, weakness, lassitude, suppressed appetite and growth, anemia, heightened risk of infection, tenderness to touch, swollen and inflamed gums, loosened teeth, swollen wrist and ankle joints, shortness of breath, fevers, petechial hemorrhages from the venules, beading or fracture of ribs at costochondral junctions, x-ray "scurvy lines" of tibia or femur, fracture of epiphysis, massive subcutaneous, joint, muscle, and intestinal hemorrhages. The overall respiratory rate is increased, despite the lassitude and weakness, and the onset of tissue changes is marked by the loss of integrity of collagen. Most of the obvious physical changes are in fact caused by the failure to maintain normal collagen.

Recent biochemical research has finally discovered the relationship between vitamin C and collagen. Collagen is unique among proteins in its high content of hydroxyproline, although proline without the hydroxyl group is a common protein constituent. Feeding hydroxyproline does not result in its use for building collagen, but after proline is built into a protein unit by the cellular ribosomes, ascorbic acid and oxygen then are essential to adding a hydroxyl group to carbon-4 of the proline to form normal collagen. In this reaction an enyzme called "collagen proline hydroxylase" serves as a catalyst (S. Udenfriend, Science 152, 1335 (1966); N. Stone and A. Meister, Nature 194, 555 (1962)). The reaction system has been demonstrated in rats, guinea pigs, and chickens. By analogy a similar mechanism is believed to explain the formation of hydroxylysine and other similar compounds such as hydroxytryptophan.

In parallel with the onset of scurvy there appears to be no change in fibrinolytic activity in the blood, but an impairment in the clotting mechanism has been reported as reflected in prolonged prothrombin time, e.g. from 20 to 40 seconds; and after administration of dicoumarol anticoagulants the contrast is much greater.

Although ascorbic acid deficiency often alters the metabolism of cholesterol in moderate degree, reports on clinical effects thus far do not establish consistant advantages (V. F. Zaitsev, A. Myasnikov, and M. B. Sheikman, Fed. Proc. 24, T 971 (1965)).

Reports on control of steroid synthesis have been very discordant also. However, injections of ACTH cause a quantitative loss of ascorbic acid from the adrenal cortex into the venous outflow, from which there is a fairly rapid recovery. Adenosinetriphosphate can induce a similar loss from the adrenal cortex. Enlargement of the adrenal glands by as much as 270 per cent during scurvy points toward a functional relationship that has not been identified.

In relation to other nutrients, ascorbic acid has been demonstrated to assist in the utilization of iron and often to afford a significant sparing or protective effect on several vitamins in the B-complex including thiamine, riboflavin, folic acid, and pantothenic acid, and on vitamins A and E (T. Terroine, Nutrio Dieta 4, 148 (1962)). The effects appear to depend on its reducing or antioxidant action. In the case of folic acid there is a conversion to the citrovorum factor. F. S. Daft et al. have shown that large intakes of ascorbic acid by albino rats can result in very marked sparing action on the requirement for several members of the vitamin B complex. The effect was found to be caused chiefly by changes in the intestinal flora, with resultant synthesis of available quantities of the B-complex vitamins. S. M. Levenson *et al.* (*Arch. Int. Med.* **110**, *693* (*1962*)) observed in studies with germfree guinea pigs on a vitamin C free diet, compared with controls in a normal environment, that their average survival was **44** days compared with **27** days for the control group. The germfree animals also grew faster, achieved higher body weight, consumed more food and showed less hemorrhage in their joints.

Moderate injections of diphtheria toxin cause losses of ascorbic acid from guinea pig glandular tissues in the range of 33 per cent; and a prior intake of the vitamin in the range of 5 to 10 mg. per day affords greater protection than lesser intakes against the resultant injury, particularly as seen in the odontoblasts and subcutaneous tissue. There is evidence of similar relationships in human experience.

People and guinea pigs on a low intake of vitamin C lose their capacity to utilize the amino acid tyrosine normally, and may excrete large amounts of an intermediate product, p-hydroxyphenylpyruvate. The deficiency appears to result from an increased activity of one enzyme leading to the pyruvate and a decrease in another that would catalyze oxidation of the pyruvate (M. N. D. Goswami and W. E. Knox, *J. Chronic Dis.* **16**, *363* (*1963*)). Earlier papers have shown many striking examples of changes in specific enzyme activities that result from low intakes of ascorbic acid.

There has been very little study of the coenzyme role of ascorbic acid in hydrolyzing mustard oil glycosides, as reported by M. D. Ettlinger and A. J. Lundeen (*J. Am. Chem. Soc.* **78**, *4172* (*1956*)).

The catabolism of ascorbic acid may lead to carbon dioxide or oxalate, or urinary excretion, depending on conditions (*Nutrition Reviews* **22**, *7* (*1964*)). There is no clear explanation concerning the losses occasioned by major surgery, bacterial toxins, or severe burns. However, some surgeons who have studied the problem suggest supplying 150 to 200 mg. per day postoperatively to restore normal blood and leucocyte values (*see Nutrition Reviews* **20**, *328* (*1962*)).

In acid products such as tomato and citrus juices the vitamin is fairly stable at room temperature, or even when heated if not contaminated by copper equipment, and it is retained normally in the range of 50 to 80 per cent in cooked, canned, frozen and freeze-dried products. The optimum dehydration for maximum stability appears to be equivalent to enough water to cover surfaces with a layer one molecule thick. Crushed or finely chopped raw vegetables generally lose their ascorbic acid content rapidly because of the air exposure and the presence of copper-protein enzymes that catalyze oxidation.

Recent studies on the oxidation of ascorbic acid and on the reduction of dehydroascorbic acid confirm the concept that there is formed a highly reactive intermediate (monodehydroascorbate) at the half-way point characterized by a free radical structure (H. S. Mason, *Ann. Rev. Biochem.* **34**, *595, 599* (*1965*)). The same intermediate has been shown to play a dominant role in the vitamin's function as a cellular respiratory catalyst (*Nutrition Reviews* **15**, *184* (*1957*)).

In view of the great number of enzymes and simpler substances that are in all living cells, many of which are reduced by ascorbic acid, and others are oxidized by the resultant dehydroascorbic acid, it is scarcely conceivable that different concentrations of the freely circulating forms of the vitamin would not cause marked changes in enzyme activity. Hence, it is not surprising that a normal range of ascorbic acid in the tissues is necessary for optimal balances and resultant health.

The above relationship has a bearing on the recommended dietary allowances for ascorbic acid. Even though about 10 mg. of ascorbic acid per day may protect a sheltered adult from scurvy for a year or two, this does not mean that the intake is anywhere near optimal. Other facts are significant. To maintain concentrations of ascorbic acid in human tissues that are in the range characteristic of persons on a mixed diet with typical quantities of fresh food, an intake in the range of 50 to 150 mg. per day is necessary. The resultant tissue storage is then within the range characteristic of nearly all animals that maintain the vitamin under physiological control and in the range of concentration found in other primates and guinea pigs on a typical mixed natural diet.

Carefully controlled tests with animals also point in the same direction. Growing guinea pigs are protected from scurvy by 0.5 mg. of ascorbic acid per day, but an intake in the range of 5.0 to 10 mg. is necessary for optimal protection against demands for reproduction and lactation, resistance to bacterial toxins, survival under stress, such as exposure to cold, infections, and severe trauma. Also, a mother on a typical mixed diet will furnish to the nursing infant about 20 to 25 mg. ascorbic acid per day, and at that level, the input maintains a normal tissue storage. In view of all the evidence at hand, the Food and Nutrition Board of the National Academy of Sci-ences-National Research Council, recommends a daily intake for normal adults of 70 mg. per day, for nursing mothers 100 mg., for infants 30 mg., and for 15-year-old adolescent children 80 mg. (*Cf. also* J. Masek, *World Rev. Nutrition Dietet.* **3,** *149 (1962)*, who suggests 80 mg. per day as a regular allowance.)

During the past 50 years, there have been many changes in the diet pattern of the United States and other Western countries. One of them has been a decreased reliance on fresh potatoes, sweet potatoes, apples, parsnips, and cabbage for supplying vitamin C, and a greater reliance on citrus fruits and juices and tomatoes. Cantaloupes and strawberries are also attractive and reliable sources, as are green peppers and broccoli. Hence, scurvy has become a rare disease and most of the population maintains a satisfactory tissue concentration (K. R. Stitt, in *Nutrition Reviews* **21,** *257 (1963)*).

The average intake per day in the United States has risen from 69 to 117 mg. However, occasional cases of scurvy occur among infants, small children, and elderly people as a result of consuming severely restricted diets. Other favorable factors have been the increased use of refrigeration, high quality canned and frozen produce, and less use of copper-containing equipment in the preparation of foods. It is fairly common practice also to add ascorbic acid to foods for purposes beyond simple nutrition, *e.g.* to protect natural flavors and colors by serving as an antioxidant.

CHAPTER XIX

PRESENT KNOWLEDGE OF VITAMIN D

GILBERT B. FORBES, M.D.

The antirachitic substance known as vitamin D is required by most vertebrate species. The vitamin can be made available to the body either as preformed vitamin D in the diet or by the action of ultraviolet light on the integumentum, a process which transforms provitamin D_3 to the active vitamin. Hence nutritional rickets is a double deficiency disease, the development of which requires the simultaneous lack of dietary vitamin D and sunlight.

Vitamin D is a very powerful substance. A daily intake of 2.5 to 10 μg. (equivalent to 100 to 400 I.U.) will prevent rickets in children, and 1 to 2 mg. daily can be toxic if continued for long periods. Chemically speaking, the provitamins ergosterol and 7-dehydrocholesterol consist of a substituted cyclopentane-perhydro-phenanthrene nucleus, and show intense absorption maxima at 271, 282, and 293 mμ. Formation of vitamin D_2 and D_3 from the respective provitamins involves the opening of ring B under the influence of ultraviolet radiation. In this process a number of other compounds with weak antirachitic properties, such as lumisterol and tachysterol, are also formed.

Ergosterol is found in certain fungi and yeasts, while 7-dehydrocholesterol occurs in animals, principally in skin and duodenal mucosa. Vitamin D as such is found in appreciable amounts only in certain fish liver oils. The method of vitamin synthesis used by the fish is not known. Other foods are rather poor sources of the vitamin: mammalian liver contains 1 to 4 I.U. per gram, egg yolk 1 to 5 I.U. per gram, and milk 3 to 100 I.U. per liter. Animals can synthesize the 7-dehydrocholesterol from cholesterol.

Many foods are now fortified with vitamin D. This is true of the vast majority of commercial milks and infant formula products; in fact the fortification of evaporated milk is required by law. There can be no doubt that the extreme rarity of infantile rickets in this country today is due in great part to the widespread fortification of milk.

Other fortified foods include some brands of margarine, cocoa, chocolate mixes, and cereals. A recent report of the Committee on Nutrition of the American Academy of Pediatrics (*Pediatrics* **31,** *512* (*1963*)) summarizes these for the U.S.A. and Canada. The estimated vitamin D intake of the modern child can vary widely; it will rarely be less than 400 I.U. per day, and may reach 2,900 I.U. in the U.S.A. and 4,100 I.U. in Canada. Obviously, the existence of food fortification must be taken into account in planning modern diets, and in coming to a decision on the need for vitamin D supplements.

One additional circumstance serves to complicate the modern scene. This is the industrial practice known as "overage." Since labeling regulations require that processed foods containing additives meet certain minimum standards, and since vitamin D slowly deteriorates on standing, some British firms are known to have added more vitamin D than is stated on the label. Whether this practice exists to any appreciable extent in the U.S.A. we do not know.

Since sunlight is antirachitic, it is impossible to set forth a dietary requirement for vitamin D without prior knowledge of the degree of exposure to sun. It is this fact which accounts for the geographic incidence of rickets, which is rare in the tropics and was formerly common in the smogbound cities of northern Europe. That it is available sunlight and not some other climatic factor which is responsible for this variation is shown by the occurrence of rickets in subtropical regions when infants are kept indoors. Rickets is a disease of growing bone, and so the need for vitamin D is related to the growth rate.

The occasional occurrence of rickets in later childhood and adolescence indicates that vitamin D is required throughout the growing period. Osteomalacia can occur in adults whose habits shield them from sunlight. The National Research Council recommends an allowance of 400 I.U. daily, as a total from all dietary sources, for infants, children, and pregnant and lactating women. In view of some studies showing that 100 to 200 I.U. suffice for the infant, this figure represents a generous margin of safety. No estimate is given for the adult allowance, and it is likely that the requirement is so small that it can be met by casual exposure to sunlight. It is well known that human rickets can be cured by repeated brief exposure to sun or artificial ultraviolet light.

The Committee on Nutrition of the American Academy of Pediatrics states its position as follows: "Thus, in the face of existing evidence, the Committee on Nutrition considers that practitioners and public health authorities should strive to ensure that the total vitamin D intake of all infants reaches the recommended allowance of 400 I.U. per day, but at the same time, they should make concerted efforts to restrict the upper limit of intake for all sources to an amount as close to this figure as practicable. This demands that cognizance be taken of the amount of vitamin D contributed by the formula and other components of the diet before prescribing a vitamin D supplement, and that attention be paid to the amount of vitamin D provided by the supplement chosen.

"It demands also, that efforts be intensified to dispel from the minds of parents the concept of vitamins as tonics.... Although there is no specific evidence that daily intakes of vitamin D in the order of 2,000 to 3,000 I.U. produce deleterious effects on individuals beyond infancy, it should be realized that the present trend in nutrition is imposing a new situation upon the children and adults of North America, the long-term effects of which are entirely unknown" (*Pediatrics* **31**, *512* (*1963*)).

There are some interesting species variations. In the chick, vitamin D_2 exhibits only one-tenth the potency of vitamin D_3. However, P. S. Chen, Jr., and H. B. Bosman (*J. Nutrition* **83**, *133* (*1964*)) have shown that this species requires a daily intake of only 6 I.U. for proper bone growth and calcium homeostasis, an amount roughly equivalent to the infant human requirement on a body weight basis. The rat is unusual in that experimental rickets is difficult to produce unless the Ca:P ratio of the diet is abnormal. The question as to why rickets fails to develop in birds and fur-bearing animals in their natural habitat is an intriguing one. It is supposed that the skin oils contain provitamin D which after activation by sunlight is ingested by licking or "preening."

Studies are now underway in a number of laboratories on the distribution and metabolism of radiolabeled vitamin D (*see* Bosmann and Chen, *Proc. Soc. Exp. Biol. Med.* **120**, *30* (*1965*)). Such studies are complicated by the fact that the active vitamin must be distinguished from degradation products which may still bear the radiolabel.

Recent investigations have quite properly focused on the mechanism of action of vitamin D. The stimulus for these studies has come from three sources: (1) the demonstration that many substances are actively transported across the gut mucosa; 2) the development of the everted gut sac technique; and 3) the demonstration that a number of substances active in trace amounts, such as hormones, exert their action by stimulating RNA synthesis.

It has been known for many years that vitamin D promotes intestinal absorption of calcium (the evidence is conflicting with regard to phosphorus); and indeed this seems to be true for most of the elements in group II of the periodic table (N. A. Worker and B. B. Migicovsky, *J. Nutrition* **75**, *222* (*1961*)). More recently, it has been shown, by the everted gut sac technique, that calcium is actively transported, that is, it moves against a concentration gradient in the intestinal wall (D. Schachter and S. M. Rosen, *Am. J. Physiol.* **196**, *357* (*1959*); H. E. Harrison and H. C. Harrison, *Ibid.* **199**, *265* (*1960*)).

Calcium transport is minimal in animals deficient in vitamin D, and is greatly enhanced by vitamin D, particularly when it is given to the intact animal prior to making the gut sac preparation. Furthermore, the vitamin D effect can be blocked by actinomycin D, a substance known to inhibit RNA synthesis.

A. W. Norman (*Am. J. Physiol.* **211**, *829* (*1966*)) has shown, in studies on ^{45}Ca absorption in the rachitic chick, that vitamin D exerts its action only after a lag period of several hours. Actinomycin D blocks the action of the vitamin only if given within three hours of the latter. Moreover, vitamin D causes a rapid increase in the pulse labeling of intestinal mucosa RNA by tritiated uridine, and this too can be inhibited by actinomycin D. R. H. Wasserman and A. N. Taylor (*Science* **152**, *791* (*1966*)) present evidence to the effect that vitamin D administration induces the formation or elaboration of a calcium binding factor by intestinal mucosa, and that this factor is a protein. Thus the evidence is consistent with the hypothesis that vitamin D acts as an initiator of enzyme synthesis in intestinal mucosa, and that these are in turn involved in the active transport of calcium.

Vitamin D may also act on the kidney. H. F. DeLuca, G. W. Engstrom, and H. Rasmussen, (*Proc. Nat. Acad. Sci.* **48**, *1604* (*1962*)) found that it affects the uptake of ^{45}Ca by kidney mitochondria. Human rickets is associated with an aminoaciduria.

It should be appreciated that large (pharmacologic) doses of vitamin D produce somewhat different effects than physiologic amounts. Both promote calcium absorption, but large doses cause bone dissolution and hypercalcemia.

Vitamin D deficiency rickets is largely a disease of the past, and increasing attention is being given to the possible harmful effects of overdosage. As mentioned previously, the American diet is generously supplied with vitamin D. There is good evidence that patients with sarcoidosis are hypersensitive to the vitamin, and as stated earlier, large doses are known to produce toxic effects in both animals and man. Epidemiologic evidence supports the contention that the mild form of the infantile hypercalcemic syndrome is the result of an excessive intake of vitamin D. In Great Britain, where a decade ago this syndrome had its highest incidence, the intake of vitamin D by infants was in the 1,000 to 4,000 I.U. range, or five to 20 times the requirement. Furthermore, most infants had been fed cows' milk, which provides about three times as much calcium as human milk (vitamin D toxicity is enchanced by high calcium intakes) and most responded satisfactorily to a diet low in calcium and vitamin D (R. G. Mitchell, *Arch. Dis. Child.* **35**, *383* (*1960*)).

On the other hand, the role of vitamin D in the severe form of the infantile hypercalcemic syndrome, which is accompanied by aortic stenosis, a peculiar facial appearance, and mental retardation, is not well established (D. Fraser, B. S. Kidd, S. W. Kooh, and L. Paunier, *Ped. Clin. N. Am.* **13**, *503* (*1966*)). These children probably suffer from some unknown congenital metabolic error. However, some do show a partial response (increased growth rate, disappearance of osteosclerosis) to a low calcium-low vitamin D diet.

Perhaps it is time that the nutritionist reexamine the basis for the vitamin D requirement, currently taken to be independent of body size, for the need for vitamin A and certain members of the B group is a function of body weight. Daily doses of 10,000 to 20,000 I.U. vitamin D taken over a period of time are intoxicating for adults (S. T. Anning, J. Dawson, D. E. Dolby, and J. T. Ingram, *Quart. J. Med.* **17,** *203* (*1948*)). This is 150 to 300 I.U. per kilogram, which suggests that, all other things being equal, 750 to 1,500 I.U. could be toxic for the 5 kg. baby. Many babies are given this much today; perhaps we should marvel not so much at the low incidence of rickets as at the rarity of apparent toxicity, a phenomenon which attests to the stamina of the modern infant.

Two recent articles are of interest. W. F. Loomis (*Science* **157,** *501* (*1967*)) discusses the role of skin pigment in the regulation of vitamin D synthesis in man. He suggests that skin color, which is known to be a function of latitude, is an adaptation which provides both for protection against rickets and minimization of excessive vitamin D synthesis in equatorial regions. H. Morii and DeLuca (*Am. J. Physiol.* **213,** *358* (*1967*)) have shown that, in contrast to parathormone, thyrocalcitonin action is independent of vitamin D.

CHAPTER XX

PRESENT KNOWLEDGE OF VITAMIN E

OSWALD A. ROELS, PH.D.

Vitamin E was discovered when male and female rats failed to reproduce normally on diets of purified fat, protein, carbohydrates, minerals, and the growth factors which were known in 1922. Addition of fresh lettuce, yeast, wheat, oats, milk fat, meat, or dried alfalfa restored normal reproductive capacity to the animals, and it was found that the restorative factor could be extracted from these foods with organic solvents. The compound was therefore classified as a fat soluble vitamin and called tocopherol.

During the past several decades, a series of compounds chemically related to vitamin E have been discovered: four naturally occurring tocopherols and their corresponding tocotrienols. All the compounds of the vitamin E series can be considered as derivatives of a hypothetical compound, 2-methyl-2-(4,8,12-trimethyltridecyl)-6-chromanol, or TOCOL:

5,8-dimethyl tocol with double bonds in the same position in the side chain or 5,8-dimethyl tocotrienol; and delta-tocotrienol is the 8-methyl tocol with double bonds between carbon atoms 3 and 4, 7 and 8, and 11 and 12 in the side chain (J. Glover, in *Biochemistry of Quinones*, R. A. Morton, Editor, p. 248. Academic Press, New York, 1965).

At present, tocopherols are isolated on a commercial scale from vegetable oils, usually by molecular distillation, extraction with organic solvents, or absorption chromatography. Alpha-tocopherol is usually the most important homologue isolated from these sources; it can also be prepared synthetically.

Alpha-tocopherol absorbed from the intestine of cannulated rats appears in the animals' lymph, indicating a lymphatic route of absorption. Vitamin E is stored in

Alpha-tocopherol is 5,7,8-trimethyl tocol, *i.e.*, the derivative with methyl groups on carbon atoms 5, 7, and 8 of the ring. Beta-tocopherol is the 5,8-dimethyl tocol; gamma-tocopherol is the 7,8-dimethyl tocol; delta-tocopherol is the 8-methyl tocol; zeta 2-tocopherol is the 5,7,8-trimethyl tocol with additional double bonds between carbon atoms 3 and 4, 7 and 8, and 11 and 12 in the side chain or 5,7,8-trimethyl tocotrienol; eta-tocopherol is the 7,8-dimethyl tocol with double bonds between carbon atoms 3 and 4, 7 and 8, 11 and 12 in the side chain or 7,8-dimethyl tocotrienol; epsilon-tocopherol has been shown to be the

the liver, and there appears to be a linear relationship between the amount of tocopherol in the diet and liver storage, although this may not hold for very high tocopherol intakes. Maximum storage occurs about six hours after administration of the vitamin. DL-Alpha-tocopherol acetate is absorbed much more slowly than the free alcohol. The bulk of the tocopherol stored in the liver cell appears to be associated with its structural parts, especially mitochondria and microsomes.

The relative biological activities of the tocopherol homologues vary greatly with chemical structure (J. Bunyan, D. McHale,

J. Green, and S. Marcinkiewicz, *Brit. J. Nutrition* **15**, *253* (*1961*)). Alpha-tocopherol is the most active biologically. Beta-tocopherol and alpha-tocotrienol have about one-third the activity of alpha-tocopherol and the other homologues exhibit relatively little biological activity.

S. R. Ames, M. I. Ludwig, D. R. Nelan, and C. D. Robeson (*Biochemistry* **2**, *188* (*1963*)) found that the isomeric acetates of 2-L-alpha-tocopherol and DL-alpha-tocopherol were 21 and 60 per cent as active respectively as D-alpha-tocopherol acetate in the resorption-gestation rat bioassay. There was no evidence of a synergistic effect of the two isomers in this biological function. Subsequently, these relative activities have been essentially confirmed with other vitamin E deficiency conditions, including encephalomalacia in the chick and dystrophy in the chick, rat, and rabbit.

A review of the biological availability of various forms of vitamin E with respect to different indices of deficiency was recently published by B. Century and M. K. Horwitt (*Fed. Proc.* **24** (*4*), *Part I, 906* (*1965*)).

I. B. Desai, C. K. Barekh, and M. L. Scott (*Biochim. Biophys. Acta* **100**, *280* (*1965*)) have shown that absorption rates for D and L epimers of alpha-tocopherol acetate from intestines of normal and dystrophic chicks are similar. The Animal Research Council sub-committee for vitamin E standards has shown that the relative potency of D-alpha-tocopherol is 1.2 times greater than that of the DL-form.

Vitamin E deficiency causes a wide variety of symptoms in different species of animals, and may affect many different tissues: as already mentioned, reproductive ability is affected in both male and female rats. The female can conceive normally, but the fetus dies and is resorbed. In the male, there is a marked atrophy of the testes, frequently resulting in sterility. In turkeys and chickens, the adverse effect of vitamin E deficiency on reproduction is a high incidence of embryonic abnormalities and mortalities,

resulting in low hatchability. The discovery that vitamin E was necessary to the house cricket (*Acheta domestica*) for normal spermatogenic activity and egg production indicates that alpha-tocopherol may be important for reproduction in widely different species.

One of the most widely occurring symptoms of vitamin E deficiency in many animals is muscular dystrophy. This has been observed in the dog, guinea pig, rabbit, chick, and *Rhesus* monkey. Whereas voluntary muscles are mainly affected in these animals, myocardial degeneration occurs in herbivorous animals.

In vitamin E deficiency, baby pigs suffer from degeneration of skeletal and cardiac muscle, degeneration of the liver, and creatinuria. Liver necrosis and muscular dystrophy do not occur in young fasting rats, but do occur in deficient rats on normal protein, low protein, or protein free diets. Nutritional muscular dystrophy also appears in infant lambs placed on a diet deficient in vitamin E. Fatal liver necrosis has developed in swine.

Neurological symptoms are observed in the chick suffering from vitamin E deficiency; encephalomalacia is common. The epithelium is also affected and massive exudative diathesis occurs.

Anemia has been observed, particularly in the *Rhesus* monkey. In this animal, skeletal muscle and bone marrow are most seriously affected. Increased erythrocyte fragility was a most significant hematological alteration in young mink deficient in alpha-tocopherol.

In human beings, it has been shown by F. Gerloczy and B. Bencze (*Acta Paediat. Hung.* **2**, *4* (*1961*)) that sclerema neonatorum (a type of edema most common in the premature human infant) can be cured by oral administration of tocopheryl acetate; vitamin E therapy reduced mortality in this disease to one-seventh. The authors found extremely low levels of tocopherol in the serum of premature infants and ascribed the therapeutic activity of vitamin E to its influence on capillary fragility.

A. S. Majaj *et al.* (*Am. J. Clin. Nutrition* **12**, *374* (*1963*)) have shown that Jordanian infants with severe kwashiorkor and macrocytic anemia and creatinuria showed positive improvement of the anemia following administration of tocopheryl phosphate and tocopheryl acetate. Urinary excretion of creatine decreased and there was a rapid increase in their reticulocytes followed by a rise in hematocrit, red blood cell count, and hemoglobin.

Horwitt (*Am. J. Clin. Nutrition* **8**, *451* (*1960*)) claims that alpha-tocopherol is important in the diet of man, and that the human requirement depends upon intake of unsaturated fatty acids. This claim was made as a result of a study on a group of adult male subjects who were put on a diet deficient in vitamin E for long periods of time. It was found that resistance of their erythrocytes to hemolysis, when incubated *in vitro* in the presence of hydrogen peroxide, was directly related to their dietary intake of alpha-tocopherol and inversely proportional to the polyunsaturated fatty acids in their diet.

It remains to be seen what is the physiological significance of decreased resistance to *in vitro* peroxide hemolysis of erythrocytes. As a result of these studies, Horwitt has recommended a daily intake of 5 mg. of alpha-tocopherol when the diet is low in unsaturated fat. When using high dietary levels of polyunsaturated fats, Horwitt recommends 30 mg. of alpha-tocopherol daily. It should be stressed here that the tocopherol content of natural oils and fats is usually proportional to their degree of unsaturation.

Very little is known about tocopherol excess in man. R. W. Hillman (*Am. J. Clin. Nutrition* **5**, *597* (*1957*)) reported that a normal adult male ingested 296 g. alpha-tocopherol over a period of 93 days, with a resulting high level in his plasma (2.26 mg. per 100 ml.). A significant but transitory creatinuria occurred during the test period, but there was no apparent change in excretion of creatine or of 17-ketosteroids. The author could not detect any signs of clinical toxicity.

J. G. Bieri, L. Teets, B. Belavady, and E. L. Andrews (*Proc. Soc. Exp. Biol. Med.* **117**, *131* (*1964*)) determined serum vitamin E levels in a normal adult urban population, and found no values below 0.5 mg. per 100 ml.; 6.1 per cent were below 0.7 mg. per 100 ml.; 70 per cent fell between 0.8 and 1.39 mg. per 100 ml., and 9.2 per cent were in the very high range. M. M. Rahman *et al.* (*Ibid.* **117**, *133* (*1964*)) examined the serum vitamin E levels in a rural Pakistani population, utilizing exactly the same technique as Bieri *et al.* In this study, 21 per cent of the sample of the population examined was found to have serum alpha-tocopherol levels below 0.5 mg. per 100 ml., and 11.2 per cent of the sample had values below 0.4 mg. per 100 ml.

It is generally difficult to compare serum tocopherol levels reported from different areas because different methods are utilized by different workers, and many determinations of this compound may be unreliable. The analytical procedure is generally based upon a colorimetric reaction depending upon the oxido-reduction potential of the samples examined. Therefore, frequently total reducing substances are measured rather than alpha-tocopherol specifically. M. Y. Dju, K. E. Mason, and L. J. Filer, Jr. (*Am. J. Clin. Nutrition* **6**, *50* (*1958*)) measured the tocopherol content of human tissues from birth to old age in necropsy samples of 70 individuals. They found that it was best to express tocopherol levels as milligrams of tocopherol per gram of fat rather than per gram of tissue.

Tocopherol levels in the lung, kidney, spleen and pancreas were of the same order as in the liver, skeletal muscle, and heart. In the pituitary, testes, and adrenals, however, levels were considerably higher. Wide variations were observed between individuals. The authors concluded that the difference in the tocopherol content of human tissues is largely caused by changes in dietary intake and absorption.

Although it is well known now that vitamin E is widely distributed in nature and that a deficiency causes a variety of symptoms in many species, its exact function at the molecular level in biological processes is not understood. Many workers have demonstrated that disease symptoms caused by its absence can be cured or prevented by a number of antioxidants. As a result, it has been suggested that the sole function of alpha-tocopherol in biological systems is that of a lipid antioxidant preventing formation of peroxides from polyunsaturated fatty acids.

Thus, H. H. Draper *et al.* (*J. Nutrition* **84**, *395* (*1964*)) found that when rats were fed a highly purified diet deficient in vitamin E the females did not reproduce. When the synthetic antioxidant N,N'-diphenyl-p-phenylenediamine (DPPD) was added to the diet at quite low levels, their normal reproductive capacity was restored. Bieri (*Biochem. Pharmacol.* **13**, *1465* (*1964*)) demonstrated that several synthetic antioxidants, fed to chicks at relatively high levels, were ineffective in preventing exudative diathesis and mortality when the diet was deficient in both selenium and vitamin E. However, when either selenite or alpha-tocopherol acetate was given with the antioxidants, deficiency signs and mortality were prevented, indicating that there is a synergistic effect between antioxidants and selenium or vitamin E.

It had been demonstrated earlier that the onset of symptoms of vitamin E deficiency in the chick could be accelerated by increasing the polyunsaturated fatty acids in the diet, and that vitamin E deficiency could be delayed in the same animal by adding some known antioxidants. Addition of DPPD does not have a sparing effect on tocopherol stored in the liver of growing rabbits and rats fed a diet deficient in vitamin

E. It has also been reported that ascorbic acid protects chicks from the characteristic lesions of vitamin E deficiency, even when they receive high dietary levels of polyunsaturated fats.

F. Christensen, H. Dam, and R. A. Gortner (*Acta Physiol. Scandinav.* **36**, *82, 87, 97* (*1956*)) believe that alpha-tocopherol may be more than just an antioxidant; synthetic antioxidants could prevent some symptoms of vitamin E deficiency in the rat and chicken, but not others. Thus, certain antioxidants could prevent encephalomalacia but not muscular degeneration in the chick. Another antioxidant could prevent muscular dystrophy but not encephalomalacia.

Interesting observations on the physiological role of vitamin E have come from J. S. Dinning, P. L. Day, and C. D. Fitch (*see Nutrition Reviews* **21**, *289* (*1963*)). These workers have studied the *Rhesus* monkey fed a diet free of tocopherol over long periods of time. They found muscular dystrophy, creatinuria, anemia, and various other hematological symptoms in their deficient animals. Pathologic lesions of skeletal muscle and bone marrow were obvious. All these symptoms could be cured and reversed by feeding alpha-tocopheryl acetate or phosphate, whereas DPPD caused only partial reversal.

The 6-chromanol of hexahydro coenzyme Q_4 also reversed all symptoms of alpha-tocopherol deficiency. The same compound cures muscular dystrophy induced in the rabbit by a diet deficient in vitamin E. The possibility remains that the preventive effect of synthetic antioxidants may result from the antioxidant protection afforded the residual stores of alpha-tocopherol. Moreover, "peroxide" levels reported in different tissues of animals deficient in vitamin E may well have been manipulative artifacts.

A series of reports has appeared from K. Schwarz and co-workers (Schwarz and C. M. Foltz, *Fed. Proc.* **19**, *421* (*1960*)) indicating that there is a complex physiological link between selenium and alpha-tocopherol. Both substances prevent exudative diathesis in the chick, but selenium does not prevent muscular dystrophy of rabbits on a diet deficient in vitamin E, nor will it prevent resorption gestation in rats. Schwarz *et al.* therefore conclude that a first group of diseases is due principally to vitamin E deficiency and may not be influenced by selenium. A second group is caused principally by selenium deficiency and is only partially affected by vitamin E, while still a third group is caused by a simultaneous lack of vitamin E and selenium: *e.g.* dietary liver necrosis in rats and multiple necrosis in the mouse.

This story was further complicated when it was shown that in certain cases amino acids containing sulfur have a sparing effect on vitamin E. It has been suggested that this is due to a possible contamination of the amino acids with selenium. However, Scott and C. C. Calvert (*J. Nutrition* **77,** *105* (*1962*)) indicated that, when chicks were fed a diet deficient in vitamin E, low dietary levels of methionine and cysteine accelerated the onset of nutritional muscular dystrophy. Adequate levels of L-cystine prevented muscular dystrophy.

A review of the biochemistry of vitamin E was published by F. D. Vasington, S. M. Reichert, and A. Nason (*Vitamins and Hormones* **18,** *43* (*1960*)) and an excellent series of review papers on vitamin E appeared in *Vitamins and Hormones* **20** (*1962*).

Since vitamin E deficiency gives rise to nutritional muscular dystrophy in many species of animals, there have been intensive investigations of the effect of alpha-tocopherol on oxidative enzyme systems. As early as 1956, J. Bouman and E. C. Slater (*Nature* **177,** *1181* (*1956*); *Biochim. Biophys. Acta* **26,** *624* (*1957*)) reported the presence of alpha-tocopherol in active respiratory enzyme systems of heart-muscle preparation.

Vasington and Nason (*Vitamins and Hormones, loc. cit.*) detected tocopherol in bovine heart NADH-cytochrome c reductase.

It was concluded from this that tocopherol may play a role in biological oxidation-reduction reactions. Indeed, Nason and I. R. Lehman (*J. Biol. Chem.* **222,** *511* (*1956*)) found a twofold to sixfold increase of NADH oxidation when alpha-tocopherol was added to partially purified particulate preparations of rat skeletal muscle; this increase was due to a restoration of cytochrome c reductase activity.

A. L. Tappel (*see Nutrition Reviews* **21,** *23* (*1963*)) has demonstrated that muscular dystrophy in rabbits deficient in vitamin E may well be due to an increased fragility of lysosomes in the affected tissues. He observed that muscle degeneration was accompanied by an increased release of a wide variety of acid hydrolases from lysosomes. These hydrolytic enzymes act on their respective substrates and cause a general breakdown of nucleic acids, proteins, carbohydrates, mucopolysaccharides, and other cell constituents. This leads to typical muscular dystrophy.

A. Guha and O. A. Roels (*Biochim. Biophys. Acta* **111,** *364* (*1965*); Roels, M. Trout, and Guha, *Biochem. J.* **97,** *252* (*1965*)) have shown that, in vitamin A deficiency, increasing doses of dietary alpha-tocopherol increase the stability of the rat liver lysosomal membrane. J. A. Lucy and J. T. Dingle (*Nature* **204,** *156* (*1964*)) have similarly demonstrated that alpha-tocopherol counteracts the lysis of rabbit erythrocytes induced by vitamin A during *in vitro* incubation.

It therefore appears that vitamin E plays an important role in insuring the stability and integrity of biological membranes. Whether this function is or is not related to its antioxidant properties remains to be seen.

Chapter XXI

PRESENT KNOWLEDGE OF BIOTIN

William F. Bridgers, M.D.

This survey, based largely upon reports published in the last decade, will of necessity be limited in scope to a few areas where our knowledge has advanced most rapidly. There is still, for example, only a paucity of information available on the pathogenesis of the various biotin deficiency syndromes. T. Terroine (*Vitamins and Hormones* **18,** *1 (1960)*) has reviewed these, including the defects in genital tract development and reproduction in biotin deficient rats; the progressive paralysis of young calves on a potassium deficient diet that is relieved by biotin excess; the kangaroo gait of the biotin deficient rat; embryonic malformations in biotin deficient chick embryos; arrest of lactation in mice and rats made biotin deficient; nervous disorders in rat, pig, chick, and man; dermatitis in mice, rats, pigs, poultry, and man; and alopecia and hair depigmentation in the rat. Insight into the causes, consequences, and possible clinical correlates of these defects will come only if nutritionists are now stimulated to study them in the light of the greatly increased knowledge of the biochemical functions of biotin.

It has long been known that a large portion of the biotin requirements of an animal may be satisfied by biosynthesis in its own intestinal flora. It is not at all uncommon to find in balance studies that the fecal content of biotin is higher than the biotin content of the diet. The use of germfree animals has strengthened this finding. For example, a germfree rat fed a biotin deficient diet loses weight, and develops alopecia and a speckled eye condition. These symptoms are reversed by an intramuscular injection of 100 μg. of biotin (P. D. Luckey *et al.*, *J. Nutrition* **57,** *169 (1955)*).

It should be mentioned that the stimulus for the suggestion that biotin was synthesized by a microorganism was that of V. du Vigneaud, K. Dittmer, E. Hague, and B. Long (*Science* **96,** *186 (1942)*). They showed that the requirement of *Corynebacterium diptheriae* for pimelic acid was satisfied with small amounts of biotin. This led ultimately to the conclusion that biotin was probably synthesized from cysteine, carbamyl phosphate, and pimelyl coenzyme A. Space does not permit a discussion of the mechanism and control of synthesis of biotin in microorganisms. The interested reader is referred to the review by T. W. Goodwin (*Biosynthesis of Vitamins and Related Compounds, p. 145. Academic Press, New York, 1963*), and work by others (A. H. Rose, M. Ilahi, and M. V. Kelemen, *Biochem. J.* **96,** *319 (1965)*; C. H. Pai and H. C. Lichstein, *Biochim. Biophys. Acta* **100,** *28, 36, 43 (1965)*).

Techniques for successful culture of mammalian cells *in vitro* now provide another valuable tool for the study of vitamin requirements under conditions that can be more precisely defined than is possible when dealing with the intact animal. In an extensive study of the nutrient requirements of certain mammalian cell lines in tissue culture, K. K. Sanford, L. T. Dupree, and A. B. Covalesky (*Exp. Cell Res.* **31,** *345 (1963)*) have demonstrated that biotin is necessary for cell survival. Interestingly, this requirement was not observed unless the vitamins in the nutrient mixture were limited to niacinamide, thiamine, riboflavin, pantothenate, choline, folate, and pyridoxal. Extensions of these studies should provide valuable insights into vitamin interrelationships.

In the last *Present Knowledge* series (*ref. bound volume of 1956*) there was a brief mention that biotin might play some essential role as a coenzyme in CO_2 fixation. Over the past ten years the elegant elucidation of this role for biotin has been a most significant advance in the field of nutrition. Many investigators made contributions, therefore this summary will cite mainly review articles on various aspects of the problem.

The work of S. Wakil and his group and of P. R. Vagelos and co-workers on the biosynthesis of saturated fatty acids has been summarized by Vagelos (*Ann. Rev. Biochem.* **33**, *139* (*1964*)). Wakil discovered that malonyl coenzyme A is an intermediate in the *de novo* synthesis of long chain fatty acids from acetyl coenzyme A. The enzyme catalyzing malonyl coenzyme A formation from acetyl coenzyme A, CO_2, and adenosinetriphosphate (ATP) is acetyl coenzyme A carboxylase. It contains biotin, and in fact this enzyme was the first one shown to contain this vitamin as its prosthetic group (Wakil and D. M. Gibson, *Biochim. Biophys. Acta.* **41**, *122* (*1960*)). Most investigators agree that this reaction is most likely the rate-determining step in fatty acid biosynthesis.

Biotin, therefore, is not only involved in the initial biosynthetic reaction leading to saturated fatty acid synthesis, but it also must play a role in the control devices used to regulate the levels of synthesis of fatty acids since, in general, regulation of a pathway is focused upon the rate limiting step. Of importance in this control is the stimulation of the carboxylation of acetyl coenzyme A by Krebs cycle intermediates. Citrate has the greatest effect (*Nutrition Reviews* **22**, *268* (*1964*)) with other intermediates, for example fumarate, showing a smaller effect. That biotin is involved in this regulation is shown by the finding that avidin, the classical biotin antagonist, totally prevents citrate activation of the carboxylase.

Further work has shown that the citrate activation is associated with a change in the physical characteristics of the enzyme itself, and that this conformational change some-

how results in stimulation of the partial reaction in which CO_2 from the CO_2-biotin-enzyme complex is transferred to acetyl coenzyme A. It is possible that biotin is involved in other ways in the regulation of fatty acid synthesis, ways as yet to be fully discovered.

All of the known biotin enzymes (acetyl coenzyme A carboxylase, beta-methylcrotonyl coenzyme A carboxylase, propionyl coenzyme A carboxylase, methylmalonyloxalacetic transcarboxylase, and pyruvate carboxylase) are transcarboxylases, all involving an acyl coenzyme A. However, biotin has also been assigned, in recent years, a role in deaminations, carbamylations, tryptophan metabolism (*Nutrition Reviews* **14**, *119* (*1956*)) purine synthesis (*Nutrition Reviews* **15**, *153* (*1957*)), protein synthesis, oxidative phosphorylation, and carbohydrate metabolism. The role of biotin in most of these reactions is unclear, but they share the feature of not being inhibited by avidin *in vitro*. It is likely, therefore, that many of the effects are indirect and that they are not due to biotin enzymes per se. For a discussion of these other roles for biotin in metabolism the reader is referred to the reviews by F. T. Mistry and K. Dakshinamurti (*Vitamins and Hormones* **22**, *1* (*1964*)) and by Terroine (*Ibid.* **18**, *1* (*1960*)).

In the case of protein synthesis, some data would suggest that there is a defect in the step involving the formation of amino acyl transfer RNA. A preparation of transfer RNA from normal rat liver will incorporate more ^{14}C-leucine than transfer RNA prepared from biotin deficient liver (Dakshinamurti and Mistry, *J. Biol. Chem.* **238**, *297* (*1963*)). It is somewhat surprising to find that it apparently is indeed the transfer RNA which is defective and not the activating enzymes. Other studies with yeast showed that, in biotin deficiency, there is an accumulation of purine precursors (F. Ahmad, A. H. Rose, and N. K. Garg, *J. Gen. Microbiol.* **24**, *69* (*1961*)), and to date the best suggestion would appear to be that there is an abnormal RNA accumulation in biotin deficient tissues, and that this RNA is probably a transfer RNA. Other experiments (Dakshinamurti and Mistry, *loc. cit.*) showed that the transfer RNA prepared from the livers of biotin deficient rats fed succinate incorporated ^{14}C-leucine equally as well as the transfer RNA from normal animals.

This suggests that the effects observed in amino acid incorporation might in part be due to a decrease in CO_2 fixation, and hence a reduction in the synthesis of dicarboxylic acids. Dicarboxylic acid synthesis would require predominantly propionyl coenzyme A carboxylase and pyruvate carboxylase, both of which are biotin enzymes. The deficiency in dicarboxylic acids would then lead to a reduction in pyruvate oxidation and tissue respiration. At this time further work is required before the importance of the two possibilities, that an abnormal transfer RNA is produced in biotin deficiency, or that there is a lack of an adequate energy supply for protein synthesis, can be assessed.

Biotin also may play some specific role in the metabolism of glucose other than in CO_2 fixation. For example, rats made biotin deficient have an impairment in the utilization of glucose. Mistry, Dakshinamurti, and V. Modi (*Arch. Biochem. Biophys.* **96**, *674* (*1962*)) confirmed earlier work of others showing that a substitution of sorbitol or fructose for glucose in biotin deficient rats improved the condition of these animals or delayed the onset of deficiency symptoms. Although some data have suggested that the block in glucose utilization is due to an impaired formation of glucose-6-phosphate, the exact nature of the defect of carbohydrate metabolism in biotin deficient animals still remains cloudy.

In a recent extension of these experiments (H. N. Bhagavan, D. B. Coursin, and Dakshinamurti, *Arch. Biochem. Biophys.* **110**, *422* (*1965*)) it was reported that ^{14}C-glucose incorporation into liver glycogen was re-duced over 90 per cent in the biotin deficient rat as compared with the normal animal. The workers attribute this to decreased activities of pyruvate carboxylase, a biotin enzyme important for active gluconeogenesis, and of phosphoenolpyruvate carboxykinase, an enzyme also known to be low in activity in biotin deficiency.

Over the last several years an area of investigation receiving more and more attention has been the interrelationships between biotin, folic acid, and vitamin B_{12}. Studies of Luckey *et al.* (*J. Nutrition* **57**, *169* (*1955*)) showed that biotin administration to rats on a diet free of biotin and folate resulted in an increase in folate excretion. It is probable that at least some of the experiments similar to these demonstrated that biotin became available to the intestinal flora that were then able to synthesize more folate. This explanation may not be entirely adequate, because in at least some studies, presumably, germfree animals were employed.

More recently a group of workers led by M. Marchetti has published a series of papers on these interrelationships. Marchetti and S. Testoni (*J. Nutrition* **84**, *649* (*1964*)) measured the effects of B_{12} administration to rats that had been on a biotin deficient regimen for 60 days. These rats showed loss of hair, growth retardation, and "spectacle eyes." All these symptoms were avoided when their diets were supplemented with 100 μg. per kilogram of B_{12} daily. Liver biotin in these B_{12} treated rats was higher than in the unsupplemented biotin deficient animals.

In companion papers (P. Puddu and Marchetti, *J. Nutrition* **84**, *255* (*1964*); *Biochem. J.* **96**, *24* (*1965*)) it was found that the livers of biotin deficient rats had a significantly higher B_{12} content than the livers of biotin deficient rats whose diets were supplemented with biotin. Uptake of oral B_{12} by major organs in the deficient animals was high, whereas absorption from the intestine and excretion were not impaired. These observations appear contradictory, since the animals on a biotin deficient diet were spared of symptoms if B_{12} was administered, yet they already had above-normal organ B_{12} levels. The suggestion is that a major defect in biotin deficiency is interference with the *utilization* of B_{12} ; or, in a sense, there is a conditioned B_{12} deficiency in the biotin deficient rat.

In other studies with biotin deficient rats, Marchetti, P. Pasquali, and L. Landi (*Biochem. J.* **94,** *763* (*1965*)) measured folate and folate coenzyme derivatives in the livers after dietary supplementation with biotin or B_{12}. Again, the levels of total liver folate-active substances were elevated after either biotin or B_{12} treatment. Additionally, the amount of citrovorum factor formed from folate by liver homogenates from biotin treated or B_{12} treated, biotin deficient animals was higher than by liver homogenates from unsupplemented biotin deficient rats.

At this point they suggest that a unitary hypothesis would be that not only B_{12} and folate, but also biotin, participate in one-carbon metabolism. The data are provocative and complicated, and perhaps do not lend themselves to as simple an explanation as is suggested above. Nonetheless, they do point to the merits of investigating vitamins and their interdependencies, very likely a fertile area for nutritionists who accept the challenge of dealing with complex interactions.

Chapter XXII

PRESENT KNOWLEDGE OF VITAMIN K

Robert E. Olson, M.D.

The molecular action of vitamin K remains an enigma to this day despite extensive work on its mode of action since its discovery by H. Dam (*Nature* **135,** *652* (*1935*)). Although there is some evidence in microorganisms that vitamin K participates in electron transport and oxidative phosphorylation, the evidence for this in higher animals is largely negative. Attempts to explain the antihemorrhagic activity of the K vitamins in mammals on the basis of a defect in electron transport or oxidative phosphorylation have not been successful. C. Martius and D. Nitz-Litzow (*Biochim. Biophys. Acta* **13,** *152* (*1954*)) suggested that the defect in prothrombin formation in vitamin K deficient chicks could be explained on the basis of a primary failure of oxidative phosphorylation which they observed in isolated mitochondria from vitamin K deficient chicks. They reasoned that the general protein synthesis might be reduced as a result of the defect in energy conservation, the more labile proteins being affected more than longer-lived proteins.

Unfortunately, the basic observation of an uncoupling of oxidative phosphorylation in liver mitochondria of vitamin K deficient or dicoumarol treated rats and chicks has not been confirmed (R. E. Beyer and E. D. Kennison, *Arch. Biochem. Biophys.* **84,** *63* (*1959*); A. M. Paolucci, P. B. R. Rao, and B. C. Johnson, *J. Nutrition* **81,** *17* (*1963*)). Neither has a reduction in ATP concentration or a maldistribution of adenine nucleotides been found in livers from deficient animals (W. D. Wosilait, *Biochem. Pharmacol.* **15,** *204* (*1966*)). Attempts to demonstrate the presence of vitamin K in the prothrombin molecule have also, thus far, been fruitless.

The great advance in our understanding of the molecular biology of protein synthesis over the past two decades (F. H. C. Crick, in *Cold Spring Harbor Symposia on Quantitative Biology* **31,** *3* (*1966*)) has led to a reappraisal of systems in which unique controls are imposed on protein synthesis. The relationship of vitamin K to the synthesis of prothrombin and three other proteins involved in the scheme of blood coagulation is an excellent model for study. In 1961, F. Jacob and J. Monod (*J. Molec. Biol.* **3,** *318* (*1961*)) proposed a hypothesis for the regulation of protein synthesis in bacteria which postulated the existence of regulatory genes responsible for the synthesis of unique regulatory proteins.

These repressor proteins were postulated to react allosterically with selected substrates and metabolites in the cell in such a way that conformational changes are produced. These, in turn, affected interaction of the protein with an operator site on the chromosome and affected the expression of biochemical information encoded in DNA. In this model, transcription of information from DNA to messenger RNA is the site of control.

The possibility that vitamin K could act as an effector in the Jacob and Monod model of control at the genetic level was explored by R. E. Olson in 1964 (*Science* **145,** *926* (*1964*)). Olson found that actinomycin D, an antibiotic which blocks DNA-dependent RNA polymerase, inhibited action of vitamin K_3 in stimulating the appearance of prothrombin in the blood of vitamin K deficient chicks over a six hour period. Subsequently, Olson (*Canad. J. Biochem.* **43,** *1565* (*1965*)) observed that the time of administration of actinomycin D prior to vitamin K affected the degree of inhibition of the action of vitamin K even though the efficacy of the block of total hepatic RNA synthesis as measured with adenine-8-^{14}C was maximal in two hours.

This raised the question of whether the obtained response to vitamin K in these chicks pretreated with actinomycin D was due to less messenger (m) RNA available for prothrombin synthesis because of decay of preformed labile messenger over the pretreatment period, or an incomplete block imposed on the relevant RNA-polymerase by the antibiotic. In a third paper (*Adv. Enzyme Reg.* **4,** *181* (*1966*)), Olson observed that puromycin was a more effective blocker of vitamin K induced prothrombin synthesis than actinomycin D in vitamin K deficient chicks. He also showed that the kinetics of the antagonism of vitamin K and dicoumarol in the control of prothrombin synthesis in the chick were consistent with an allosteric interaction of the two compounds with a single protein.

B. C. Johnson, R. B. Hill, R. Alden, and G. S. Ranhotra (*Life Sci.* **5,** *385* (*1966*)) reported similar experiments in vitamin K deficient and warfarin treated rats. In their experiments, actinomycin D reduced the amount of "one-stage" prothrombin stimulated by vitamin K$_1$ administered at various intervals up to five hours after the antibiotic was given, but not the rate of appearance of the protein. Puromycin and cycloheximide, another blocker of mRNA translation, were more effective in antagonizing the action of vitamin K$_1$ in these rats. These workers concluded that vitamin K was probably working at the translational level and speculated that it could be effective in removing a "properly folded structure" from the ribosomes.

J. W. Suttie (*Arch. Biochem. Biophys.* **118,** *166* (*1967*)) reported that proconvertin (Factor VII) activity could be detected in the perfusate of a rat liver treated *in vitro* with vitamin K$_1$. This effect was nullified by puromycin but not by actinomycin

D. H. Prydz (*Scandinav. J. Clin. Lab. Invest.* **17,** *143* (*1965*)) made similar observations of the effect of vitamin K and puromycin on Factor VII elaboration by liver cell suspensions. In contrast, B. M. Babior (*Biochim. Biophys. Acta* **123,** *606* (*1966*)) found that Factor VII formation, stimulated *in vivo* by intravenous vitamin K$_1$ in rats, continued apace *in vitro* in surviving liver slices in the presence of puromycin. J. P. Olson, L. L. Miller, and S. B. Troup (*J. Clin. Invest.* **45,** *690* (*1966*)), observed only miniscule effects of puromycin upon the formation of prothrombin (Factor II), Stuarts factor (Factor X), and Factor VII in the perfused rat liver.

These confusing results, supporting only in part the long accepted postulate that vitamin K stimulates *de novo* coagulation proenzyme synthesis, must be viewed against the elegant immunofluorescence studies by M. I. Barnhart and G. F. Anderson (*Biochem. Pharmacol.* **9,** *23* (*1962*)) showing that the dicoumarol treated dog shows no evidence of prothrombin in his hepatic parenchymal cells and that it appears promptly in the endoplasmic reticulum of these cells after administration of vitamin K$_1$ prior to its appearance in the plasma.

As regards the "active" form of vitamin K in animal tissues, it seems likely that multiple forms derived both from the diet and from *de novo* alkylation of 2-methyl-1,4 naphthoquinone (menadione) *in vivo* stimulate prothrombin synthesis in the liver of mammals and birds. Martius and H. O. Esser (*Biochem. Z.* **331,** *1* (*1958*)) first showed that menadione is converted to vitamin K$_{2(20)}$ in the chick, a finding which has been confirmed in this laboratory and elsewhere (P. Griminger and G. Brubacher, *Poultry Sci.* **45,** *512* (*1966*)). The yield, however, is low, the major metabolites being the glucuronide and sulfate of reduced menadione (R. Losito, C. A. Owen, Jr., and E. V. Flock, *Biochemistry* **6,** *62* (*1967*)).

This alkylation of menadione by geranyl-

geranyl-pyrophosphate appears to be rate limiting in the physiological response of animals to this unnatural vitamin. On the other hand, the proposition advanced by the Martius group (M. Billeter, W. Bolliger, and Martius, *Biochem. Z.* **340**, *290* (*1964*)) that all dietary homologues of vitamin K were dealkylated by intestinal bacteria, absorbed as menadione, and realkylated *in vivo* to vitamin $K_{2(20)}$ does not appear to be true. J. T. Matschiner, W. V. Taggart, and J. M. Amelotti (*Biochemistry* **6**, *1243* (*1967*)) have shown that the principal form of vitamin K in beef liver is a very long chain homologue more lipophilic than vitamin $K_{2(50)}$. This vitamer is apparently made in the rumen by bacteria, absorbed, and stored in the liver where it is fully functional as determined by bioassay.

In summary, it may be stated that the lipophilic quality of naturally occurring forms of vitamin K is required for their biological activity. The rapidity of action of menadione appears to be related to the rate of its conversion to such lipophilic forms by alkylation in the animal body. It is suggested that both vitamin K and the coumarin anticoagulant drugs combine allosterically with a regulatory protein and thus modify its conformation. The discovery by R. A. O'Reilly *et al.* (*New Engl. J. Med.* **271**, *809* (*1964*)) of a kindred with genetically determined resistance to the anticoagulant action of the coumarin drugs, yet possessing a normal drug metabolism, suggests that the binding sites for coumarin drugs on their regulatory protein were of low instead of high affinity. Sensitivity to vitamin K was normal in this group.

The present evidence would favor the view that the action of vitamin K is mediated via a regulatory protein at the translational stage in protein synthesis, *i.e.*, at the polysomal level. The model proposed by A. L. Cline and R. M. Bock (*Cold Spring Harbor Symposia on Quantitative Biology* **31**, *321* (*1966*)), which provides for allosteric combination of nascent peptide with regulatory proteins as an aid to their release from the ribosome, is an attractive one for the control of coagulation proenzyme synthesis by vitamin K. The similarity in the physical-chemical properties of these four clotting proenzymes, *i.e.*, prothrombin, plasma thromboplastin component, proconvertin, and Stuarts factor, which could provide a common binding site for a regulatory protein, is additional suggestive evidence for the validity of this model.

Chapter XXIII

PRESENT KNOWLEDGE OF NIACIN

Olaf Mickelsen, Ph.D.

Before 1955, primary emphasis relative to the vitamin niacin was its role as a nutrient. Since then, attention has shifted, to a certain extent, to the pharmacological field. This shift occurred when it was noted that ingestion of 4 g. niacin by human subjects produced an 11 per cent reduction in serum cholesterol levels. The reduction was proportional to initial serum cholesterol levels, since patients with levels greater than 250 mg. per 100 ml., when given a 1 g. dose of niacin, showed a 22 per cent reduction (for review, see *Niacin in Vascular Disorders and Hyperlipemia*, R. Altschul, Editor. *Charles C Thomas, Springfield, Illinois, 1964*).

Niacin therapy appears to be effective for a number of years (N. A. Christensen, R. W. P. Achor, K. G. Berge, and H. L. Mason, *Dis. Chest.* **46**, *411* (*1964*); M. L. Stern, *Current Therap. Res.* **7**, *195* (*1965*)), and in about 80 per cent of the patients. The amount of niacin required to reduce blood cholesterol levels is several hundredfold greater than the daily vitamin requirement.

Large doses reduce not only free and esterified cholesterol in the blood but also the beta-lipoproteins and triglycerides (O. N. Miller, J. G. Hamilton, and G. A. Goldsmith, *Am. J. Clin. Nutrition* **8**, *480* (*1960*); J. R. Shawver, J. S. Scarborough, and S. M. Tarnowski, *Am. J. Psychiat.* **117**, *741* (*1961*)). The latter are reduced to as great an extent as the cholesterol.

Large doses of niacin may influence lipid metabolism by inhibiting free fatty acid (FFA) mobilization from adipose tissue. Niacin inhibits release of FFA in subjects while resting and also during exercise (L. H. Carlson and L. Oro, *J. Atherosclerosis Res.* **5**, *436* (*1965*)).

The large doses necessary to reduce blood cholesterol levels have been associated with a number of disturbing side reactions. Earliest and most prominent is flushing of the skin, with a concomitant itching and feeling of heat. After a few days to a week, this phenomenon either subsides or becomes tolerable (*see Niacin in Vascular Disorders and Hyperlipemia, p. 50*). Cessation of niacin therapy for only three days results in a repetition of the flushing reaction when therapy is resumed.

Other complaints include gastrointestinal irritation with anorexia, nausea, vomiting, and diarrhea. These appear to become more prominent after three years of therapy. Liver damage associated with niacin therapy involved alterations in the following tests arranged in order of decreasing frequency: cephalin-cholesterol flocculation, serum glutamic oxalacetic transaminase, sulphabromphthalien retention, and increased serum alkaline phosphatase (Christensen, *loc. cit.*).

None of these indicated any severe degree of liver disturbance, and, in most cases, the abnormality disappeared within a short while after therapy was stopped. The significance of these mild liver disturbances is open to question since there has been no "consistent pattern of abnormality in hepatic biopsies in patients with abnormal function studies" (W. B. Parsons, *in Niacin in Vascular Disorders and Hyperlipemia, p. 263*). Fasting blood sugar levels show a variable response to high intakes of niacin.

One investigator (W. B. Parsons, Jr., *J.*

Am. Med. Assn. **173,** *1466* (*1960*)) reported that seven patients receiving niacin therapy showed "evidence of activation of peptic ulcers, with occult bleeding in one." All these patients either had ulcers earlier or were "tense, high-strung" indivduals and for these reasons niacin "was certainly not the sole factor responsible for the development of ulceration and, indeed, may have played a minor role." In another long-term study there were no signs of peptic ulcers "and the two persons with previously known duodenal ulcers experienced no exacerbation of symptoms during therapy with nicotinic acid" Berge *et al., Am. J. Med.* **31,** *24* (*1961*)).

There seems reasonable agreement that, by the oral route, niacin is effective in lowering serum cholesterol levels while niacinamide is ineffective. The situation may be different when these compounds are given by injection (R. Fontenot, H. Redetzki, and R. Deupree, *Proc. Soc. Exp. Biol. Med.* **119,** *1053* (*1965*)).

The action of niacin on animals' plasma cholesterol levels has been studied in the rabbit, rat, and dog. In the rabbit, large oral doses of niacin result in a quick reduction of cholesterol levels. Contrary to the situation in man, the reduction was not proportional to the control level.

Not only does niacin appear to keep serum cholesterol levels of rabbits fed cholesterol close to normal, but it seems to maintain a normal composition of their aortas (J. M. Murrill and J. Lemley-Stone, *Circulation Res.* **5,** *617* (*1959*)), and also is partially successful in inhibiting excess cholesterol deposition in the liver. There is some evidence that in rabbits niacin is effective in preventing any great extension of plaques but has little effect on those that may be present when therapy is started (P. Lipton and J. G. Michels, *Geriatrics* **20,** *379* (*1965*)).

In the rat, it is difficult to elevate serum cholesterol above 80 mg. per 100 ml. unless dietary cholesterol is combined with bile salts and a thyroid depressant. Even when cholesterol levels in rats were increased, addition of either 0.2 or 1.0 per cent niacin to the ration had no effect (J. L. Gaylor, R. W. F. Hardy, and C. A. Baumann, *J. Nutrition* **70,** *293* (*1960*)). Liver cholesterol levels were not influenced by either niacin (C. H. Duncan and M. M. Best, *J. Lipid Res.* **1,** *159* (*1960*)), or its amide (Gaylor, Hardy, and Baumann, *loc. cit.*).

In a sense, the dog is almost as resistant to experimentally induced atherosclerosis as the rat. This may partially explain why the dog also appears to be immune to the effect of niacin as far as cholesterol levels are concerned.

In one report, niacin at daily levels of 200 mg. per kilogram body weight had no influence on dogs' plasma cholesterol levels (M. E. Zanetti and D. M. Tennent, *Proc. Soc. Exp. Biol. Med.* **112,** *991* (*1963*)). Niacinamide at the same dose level increased cholesterol levels in normal and hypercholesteremic dogs. A final note of confusion was provided by a report that 50 mg. niacin given by mouth to dogs reduced blood cholesterol levels (F. Comesana, A. Nara, B. L. Fishleder, and D. Sodi-Pallares, *Am. Heart J.* **55,** *476* (*1958*)). One can only conclude that the effect of niacin on the blood cholesterol level of dogs has not been established.

Poultry appear to show no prominent response to niacin therapy when fed rations containing cholesterol.

It is impossible to determine whether niacin therapy has been effective in reducing or checking the atherosclerotic process in man. There appears to be ample evidence that lower serum cholesterol levels following niacin therapy are associated with a reduction in the size of xanthomas containing lipids. Although fairly large numbers of patients with signs of cardiovascular disease have been treated with niacin, therapeutic protocols have varied to such an extent that it is impossible to reach a conclusion about the efficacy of the treatment.

In recent years, the primary emphasis on niacin in grains has been on attempts to isolate the "bound" form in corn and other cereal products. This work was initiated by the observation that there was a marked difference in values for niacin in cereals as determined by a colorimetric method before and after hydrolysis with dilute sodium hydroxide. Microbiological assays indicated about 20 per cent more niacin in dilute alkaline extracts of wheat than in water or acid extracts. The substance which, on treatment with alkali, was converted to a compound with niacin activity was designated the niacin "precursor." It is very likely that the "precursor" is the same substance as the "bound" niacin investigated by subsequent workers.

Later work indicated that bound niacin in cereals was ineffective in curing the niacin deficient rat, chick, duck, and pig. Evidence for the availability of bound niacin for human subjects is not as clear-cut as that for animals.

Since the bound form is unavailable for growth of microorganisms, assay of foods before and after treatment with sodium hydroxide has been used as a measure of bound niacin. These assays indicate that 80 to 90 per cent of the niacin in such cereals as rice, wheat, corn, and barley is in the bound form. Legumes and animal products contain no bound niacin.

Attempts to isolate the bound form resulted in identification of two major kinds of compounds. One appeared to be primarily peptides with molecular weights of 12,000 to 13,000. These compounds were called niacinogens. Other workers reported isolation of a carbohydrate complex (molecular weight 2,370) as bound niacin, and felt the 2 per cent amino acids represented a protein impurity. They proposed the name niacytin for the compound (*Nutrition Reviews* **19**, *242* (*1961*)).

The existence of two different types of

bound niacin compounds leaves a number of unanswered questions. Apparently work has come to a standstill just when the problem was becoming exciting.

From a practical standpoint, some reference should have been made to the bound form of niacin when the *Recommended Dietary Allowances* were published with the term "niacin equivalents" replacing "niacin" (*National Academy of Sciences— National Research Council publication 589, p. 14. Washington, D. C., 1958*). Values for the distribution of niacin in foods have been presented, completely ignoring the bound form of niacin (B. K. Watt and A. L. Merrill, *U. S. Department of Agriculture Handbook No. 8, 1963*).

Only partial explanations are available for the poor attention bound niacin has received. Many investigators assume that the maximum value for the niacin content of a food is the correct one—presumably lower values are indicative of incomplete extraction or some analytical difficulty. There is still some disagreement as to the influence of food preparation on the availability of bound niacin, with some investigators arguing that boiling corn makes the niacin available.

In 1960, a report suggested that pellagra could develop in people who consumed large amounts of millet (*Sorghum vulgare* or jowar). On the basis of this study, it was suggested that jowar produces pellagra, not by a deficiency of tryptophan or poor availability of its nicotinic acid, but by its high content of leucine. The original work was later retracted (*see Nutrition Reviews* **21**, *334* (*1963*)).

Despite this retraction, the investigators now claim that a supplement of 10 g. L-leucine per day for five days decreased by one-half the ability of red cells to synthesize nicotinamide nucleotides when incubated with niacin (N. Raghuramulu, S. G. Srikantia, B. S. Narasinga Rao, and C. Gopalan, *Biochem. J.* **96**, *837* (*1965*)). There were, however, no differences in the levels of nucleotide in the red cells secured from 47 normal subjects and 25 pellagrins either before or after the leucine ingestion.

The extension of these studies to weanling rats (Raghuramulu, Narasinga Rao, and Gopalan, *J. Nutrition* **86**, *100* (*1965*)) suggested that adding leucine to an 11 per cent casein ration increased urinary excretion of quinolinic acid. Excretion of quinolinic acid was only partially reduced by adding 1 mg. niacin per 100 g. ration and not at all by 100 mg. DL-tryptophan. Whether leucine affects niacin is doubtful; but if it does, it did not reduce body weight gains of the rats in the preceding study.

The work with millet or jowar, if it can be repeated, appears more important. According to B. Belavady and Gopalan (*Lancet* **2**, *1220* (*1965*)), jowar contains large amounts of niacin, presumably available to animals. Furthermore, the tryptophan content "unlike that of maize, is not low." In spite of the high nutritive value of millet, it appears to cause pellagra in human subjects and blacktongue in dogs.

Tryptophan can serve as a precursor for niacin for most animals and man. The fact that the concentration of these two compounds in foods varies and their nutritional availability may differ poses a number of problems in evaluating the niacin equivalent of foods. Despite these difficulties, there appears to be increasing acceptance that approximately 60 mg. dietary tryptophan equal 1 mg. niacin insofar as vitamin requirements are concerned.

As to availability of tryptophan for niacin formation, there is relatively little experimental evidence, most of it with rats. These results do not always agree with other observations. Part of the difficulty arises from the assumption that excretion of urinary compounds related to niacin metabolism can serve as an index of the extent to which tryptophan can replace niacin. That such an assumption is not necessarily valid was apparent in some of the early work in this area.

No comprehensive investigation has been made of the efficacy of free tryptophan versus that in casein and other proteins in preventing a niacin deficiency and the relation thereof to the excretion of niacin metabolites.

In human subjects, conversion of tryptophan to niacin has been evaluated primarily by excretion of N′-methylnicotinamide (NMN) and its pyridone (either the 2 or 6 carbon in the pyridine ring has an oxygen attached to it). Many investigators observed that when diets of adults were supplemented with niacin, niacinamide, or tryptophan, urinary excretion of NMN or its pyridone increased. However, the relative contribution of these two compounds varies. One group of investigators reported that when niacinamide was given adults, the increase in pyridone excretion accounted for 70 to 90 per cent, while the NMN accounted for 10 to 30 per cent (G. A. Goldsmith, O. N. Miller, and W. G. Unglaub, *J. Nutrition* **73**, *172* (*1961*)). If other urinary compounds were measured, the results might be different.

Depending on the criteria used in estimating the extent of conversion, different values are likely to be secured. Suggestive evidence for this comes from the observation that when tryptophan in a semipurified diet just met minimal requirements, 5 mg. niacin were required to maintain nitrogen equilibrium; 10 mg. were needed to bring blood pyridine nucleotides to normal (V. M. Vivian, R. R. Brown, J. M. Price, and M. S. Reynolds, *J. Nutrition* **88**, *93* (*1966*)).

That a considerable amount of niacin is formed from dietary tryptophan is suggested by the fact that in a group of normal adult males, urinary excretion of NMN and pyridone exceeded the niacin in the diet (D. J. de Lange and C. P. Joubert, *Am. J. Clin. Nutrition* **15**, *169* (*1964*)). This could be interpreted to mean that about two-thirds of the niacin metabolized by adults fed a good diet is derived from tryptophan.

Excretion of pyridone and NMN may be

influenced by the type of protein in the diet and the physiological condition of the subject (pregnancy and acute starvation). During the third trimester of pregnancy, women excreted three times more pyridone and NMN than three months postpartum (A. E. Wertz, M. E. Lojkin, B. S. Bauchard, and M. B. Derby, *J. Nutrition* **64,** *339* (*1958*)). There is no explanation for the apparently larger stores of niacin in pregnant women. The opposite would have been anticipated, since in the third trimester the foetus grows very rapidly. Formation of new body tissue should reduce niacin stores in the mother rather than increasing them to the extent represented by the threefold greater excretion of niacin metabolites.

Little attention has been given to excretion of niacin metabolites during periods of starvation. One study in which young women were fed a semipurified diet containing different levels of niacin and tryptophan produced urinary excretion data which were interpreted as indicating that conversion of tryptophan to niacin was not altered during periods of restricted protein synthesis (Vivian, *J. Nutrition* **82,** *395* (*1964*)).

However, dietary conditions were changed every six days. Six days may be too soon to develop a state of equilibrium.

Early work on niacin excretion in acute starvation was performed before recognition of NMN and pyridone. At that time it was reported that large increases in urinary niacin occurred in dogs and normal men when no food was consumed.

Animal experiments provide evidence more divergent than that from human studies. The rat, which has been most used, is relatively resistant to niacin deficiency and diverse dietary conditions are encompassed by these studies. These conditions may exert a pronounced influence on the intestinal flora of these animals, with subsequent nutritional repercussions.

A number of investigators have concluded that, in the rat, tryptophan is first used to establish nitrogen equilibrium, then for growth, and only thereafter is it converted to niacin.

The equivalency of tryptophan to niacin varies not only from individual to individual but also with the diet, the individual's condition, and the criteria used. Some evidence suggests that interindividual variability in niacin formation from tryptophan becomes greater as the level of dietary tryptophan is increased. This variability was seen not only in adults (M. K. Horwitt *et al.*, *J. Nutrition*, **60,** *Suppl. 1* (*1956*) ; Goldsmith, Miller, and Unglaub, *Ibid.* **73,** *172* (*1961*)) but also among young girls (E. Z. Moyer, Goldsmith, Miller, and J. Miller *Ibid.* **79,** *423* (*1963*)). Results of all these studies suggest that, for good diets, an average of 60 mg. tryptophan is converted to 1 mg. niacin. When diets contain large amounts of gelatin, more tryptophan is required. In the latter situation, amino acid imbalance was given as the explanation.

The amount of tryptophan required to synthesize 1 mg. niacin appears to be reduced in pregnant women. During the third trimester, increased excretion of niacin metabolites was interpreted as indicating that only 18 mg. tryptophan were required (Wertz *et al.*, *loc. cit.*). Even three months postpartum, the continued high excretion of niacin metabolites suggested that an average of 31 mg. was needed.

When the increase in blood pyridine nucleotides was used as the measure of equivalency, a single dose of 5 g. tryptophan produced the same change as 1 g. niacin (M. Duncan and H. P. Sarett, *J. Biol. Chem.* **193,** *317* (*1951*)). These results are in line with those seen when the increase in liver pyridine nucleotides was measured in rats following large intakes of tryptophan or niacin (M. A. Morrison, M. S. Reynolds, and A. E. Harper, *J. Nutrition* **80,** *441* (*1963*)).

CHAPTER XXIV

PRESENT KNOWLEDGE OF PANTOTHENIC ACID

WILLIAM B. BEAN, M.D.

In the last decade study of pantothenic acid has been creeping forward rather than advancing with rapidity. Work on pantothenic acid has not been active. For instance, in 1964 and 1965 it does not appear in the index of *Nutrition Reviews*. The term pantothenic acid comes from the Greek word which means "from everywhere." The vitamin permeates almost any natural diet. Spontaneous deficiency of pantothenic acid is unlikely in nature since in a diet deficient in pantothenic acid the limiting and lethal deficiencies of other vitamins create their havoc first. The long and arduous as well as expensive studies necessary in man are wearisome and frustrating, so progress has been meager.

The story of the discovery of pantothenic acid reveals that it was the outcome of years of research on the "bios" effect of yeast, the chick "antipellagra factor," the filtrate "antidermatitis factor" for chicks, and a growth factor for lactic acid bacteria. Finally, all turned out to be the same thing. R. J. Williams and his collaborators continued to do basic work during the critical early years of its isolation, identification, and final synthesis. The pantothenic acid molecule is composed of beta-alanine and hydroxydimethyl-butyrolactone.

For a period of nearly 15 years, we have been experimenting with volunteers in an effort to produce an isolated deficiency of pantothenic acid without other deficiencies of essential food factors, as well as combined deficiencies. We have employed a purified, partly synthetic diet, with or without the pantothenic antagonists, such as omega-methyl-pantothenic acid. Anything like a natural diet is out of the question because of the occurrence of significant amounts of

pantothenic acid in such a wide variety of foods. Furthermore, some tests indicate that in a good many samples of food the pantothenic acid content was higher than that listed in available tables.

In 1962, we reported studies on six volunteer subjects who were investigated to find out whether immunologic responses differed in those deficient in pantothenic acid from responses in subjects given an adequate diet (*Am. J. Clin. Nutrition* **10,** *500, 506* (*1962*); *Ibid.* **11,** *85, 180, 187* (*1962*)). The control subjects remained well throughout the 13 week study. Those with a deficient diet alone had some malaise and vomiting during the third and fourth weeks and one continued to have abdominal distress and burning cramps, but repeated examination failed to disclose any objective sign. Later, tenderness in the heels, fatigue, and insomnia occurred.

The two men who received the deficient diet plus omega methyl pantothenic acid had similar symptoms which began earlier: pain and soreness in the abdomen, frequent nausea, occasional regurgitation of formula, some personality changes, perhaps related to insomnia, weakness and cramps in the legs, and paresthesias in the hands and feet. The tendon reflexes remained normal. There were intermittent but never major attacks of diarrhea. The eosinopenic response to ACTH was impaired and the sedimentation rate became elevated.

Total serum nitrogen remained unchanged. There was a slight decrease in the concentration of gammaglobulin in the subjects receiving the deficient diet with or without the antagonist. Immunization with the antigens of typhoid, Asian influenza, and tetanus induced the following reactions.

There was no difference in response to typhoid. Those deficient in pantothenic acid produced less antibody against tetanus than did the control subjects or the deficient ones who got the antivitamin. The results of the Asian flu studies were indeterminate.

Heterologous skin grafts were accepted poorly by the deficient subjects and did not proliferate well. They were rejected at least as rapidly as in the control subjects. Whether this was hastened by the secondary infection or was related to poor wound healing cannot be decided. It is possible that omega methyl pantothenic acid acted as a vitamin in the production of antibodies against tetanus.

A comparison study of pyridoxine indicated that, although a clinical illness was produced by a deficient diet and deoxypyridoxine, there was very slight impairment of the formation of antibodies against tetanus and typhoid in the deficient subjects.

A further study, however, with combined pyridoxine and pantothenic acid deficiencies had the following results. When just the diet was deficient, there was no impairment of antibody production in seven weeks. In five subjects given a diet deficient in pantothenic acid and pyridoxine with omega methyl pantothenic acid plus deoxypyridoxine all became ill. They were completely unable to respond to tetanus and to typhoid "O" antigen and had an insignificant response to typhoid "H" antigen. After restoration of the vitamins to their diet, responses in antibody formation were normal. By contrast, all five deficient men had excellent responses to immunization with poliomyelitis antigens. The serum protein fraction showed a significant decline in the amount of gammaglobulin and this paralleled the titer in typhoid "O" antibodies.

Other studies indicate that, in germfree animals, practically all the pantothenic acid fed or originally present can be accounted for by measuring the excreta and evaluating the quantity in the carcass. Thus it appears that pantothenic acid is not significantly metabolized or broken down in germfree rats (*Nutrition Reviews* **14**, *116* (*1956*)).

It was demonstrated that young rats deprived of pantothenic acid gradually lose their natural species resistance to *corne-bacterium* 197 (*Nutrition Reviews, loc. cit.*). There is considerable variation among different strains of animals and from species to species (*Ibid.* **14**, *92* (*1956*)).

A. E. Axelrod and co-workers have demonstrated convincingly that pantothenic acid deficiency impaired the production of hemagglutinating antibodies and of antibodies to diphtheria toxoid, but did not cause a reduction in the level of complement. It is not known whether the effect is produced by changing the metabolism of the antigen, damaging the cells which manufacture antigen, depressing essential enzyme systems, increasing the destruction or elimination of antibody, or something else (*see Nutrition Reviews* **14**, *150* (*1956*)).

W. J. Griffiths and his associates have demonstrated that rats required to run on a treadmill on alternate days select increasing amounts of calcium pantothenate during the exercise periods. Whether pantothenic acid changed the taste of the water or whether this was in response to an increased physiological need could not be answered by the experiments (*see Nutrition Reviews* **15**, *58* (*1957*)).

It appears that pantothenic acid is necessary as a supplement for swine fed a soybean ration as the major source of protein, although further work is needed (*Nutrition Reviews* **15**, *275* (*1957*)).

Emphasis in biochemistry has been shifting away from animals to parts of animals and away from organs to cells, to cell fractions and their highly purified enzyme systems. No one denies that information obtained by studying such systems is fundamental in research and is helpful in understanding many nutritional problems. But new ideas must continue to be fed in from observations on man and on animals. There is continuing need for this type of study.

The work of T. F. Zuker and his colleagues on the induction of severe duodenal ulcer in certain lines of experimental rats by inducing a deficiency of pantothenic acid is a good illustration of the kind of clue that may come from properly conducted studies. Its significance in human peptic ulcer is a matter of speculation. There is a very wide variation in susceptibility among different strains of rats. Acetylcholine synthesis did not seem to be affected.

The weight of the thymus gland decreased rapidly under the influence of pantothenic acid deficiency. This response could be prevented by adrenalectomy. Further studies indicated that the thymus, itself, was more susceptible to adrenal cortical hormones which were not overproduced. The development of duodenal ulcer was associated with an increase in secretion of hydrochloric acid which occurred in adult animals, not in young or growing ones (see Nutrition Reviews 17, 27 (1959)).

Administration of omega-methyl-pantothenic acid to rats impairs production of corticosterone by the adrenal glands (Nutrition Reviews 18, 273 (1960)). Deficient rats excreted only about half as much corticosterone. This could be corrected by injecting the active vitamin 24 hours before tests were made. Deficient animals could respond to ACTH.

Hepatic insulinase is diminished in rats deficient in pantothenic acid. Similar effects are produced by the deficiencies of protein or riboflavin but not deficiencies of thiamine (Nutrition Reviews 18, 93 (1960)).

Many studies have not yet revealed exactly how large doses of ascorbic acid will prevent the development of symptoms of pantothenic acid deficiency in growing rats. It is thought that this occurs through an effect on the microflora of the gut, though evidence is not final. The anemia which may occur in animals deficient in pantothenic acid may in part be explained by the finding that the synthesis of amino-levulinic acid requires both pantothenic acid and pyridoxine. Thus, this precursor of heme is specifically influenced by adequate supplies or deficiency of pantothenic acid.

In ducklings deficient in pantothenic acid there is a severe depression of the capacity to incorporate glycine and succinate into heme, and this effect may be noted in less than three days after the deficient diet is introduced. The incorporation of amino-levulinic acid was not observed until the sixth day. Addition of coenzyme A to the incubation mixtures was without effect, but calcium pantothenate injected into deficient birds only one hour before the blood samples were removed showed that glycine could be incorporated into heme at the usual rate (Nutrition Reviews 16, 142 (1958)).

Detailed studies on the food requirements of Chinook salmon have indicated that pantothenic acid is essential for their proper growth, development, and well-being; that its deficiency is characterized by clubbed gills, exudate on the gills, prostration, loss of appetite, and general sluggishness. There was no clear description of how one diagnoses prostration in a small growing salmon, but no doubt they seemed tired (Nutrition Reviews 16, 106 (1958)).

Pyridoxine or pantothenic acid deficiency rendered rats unable to respond with normal antibody formation when challenged by an influenzal vaccine. Thiamine had no effect (Nutrition Reviews 19, 116 (1961)). In guinea pigs, omega-methyl-pantothenic acid has been very effective in producing pantothenic acid deficiency, which is characterized by rather extensive reduction in serum ascorbic acid (Ibid. 19, 156 (1961)). In healthy rats pantothenic acid is rather freely distributed in the adrenal cortex. After stimulation with ACTH the concentration of coenzyme A increases selectively in the zona fasciculata at the expense of free pantothenic acid (*Ibid.* **19,** *79 (1961)*). Pantothenic acid is unstable to heat and in heat dried and in canned and in cooked meats there may be losses ranging from 15 to 30 per cent (*Ibid.* **20,** *257 (1962)*).

Pantothenic acid, although widely rumored to have an ameliorating effect on ileus and less severe reductions of function of the alimentary canal, particularly after surgical operations, has been found to have no evident effect. The reports suggesting that it did have some effect were notable for their poor controls.

Feeding pregnant rats a diet deficient in pantothenic acid produces a variety of congenital defects in the offspring. The specific defects depend on the stage of pregnancy when the diet was fed and the length of the deficiency period. The time just before birth witnesses a great increase in fetal guinea pig CoA and pantothenate, suggesting that there might be a critical need at this time. The survival time in pregnant guinea pigs was only half of that of the nonpregnant

controls, or of male guinea pigs on the same deficient diet.

In nearly all the animals hemorrhages occurred in the adrenals, and gastrointestinal hemorrhages in about one-fourth. Liver CoA and pantothenic acid fell by 50 per cent. When the deficient diet was fed through the sixth or seventh week of gestation, no harm was done, but giving the deficient diet during the ninth week caused abortions, fetal death, and death of one pregnant guinea pig. When the deficient diet was fed during the tenth week the effects were much less severe or critical. Guinea pigs have a higher requirement for pantothenic acid than do rats, in which deficiencies for a whole month during gestation have not been found to produce serious ill effects (*Nutrition Reviews* **24,** *169 (1966)*).

In conclusion, the last decade has not been a period of intensive or extensive work on pantothenic acid. The results obtained are significant, though not numerous. Much more study is needed.

CHAPTER XXV

PRESENT KNOWLEDGE OF FOLACIN

JOSEPH J. VITALE, PH.D.

Folacin (folic acid, folate, or pteroylglutamic acid (PGA)) is a synthetic product and not usually found in nature; it is usually conjugated with two or six molecules of glutamic acid which are linked at the gamma-carbon positions. The physiologically active form is a reduction product (*Figure 1*), 5, 6, 7, 8-tetrahydrofolic acid (THF) linked in the 5_N, 10_N, or 5_N–10_N positions with formyl, hydroxymethyl, methyl, or formimino groups.

the oxidized form or the reduced folate form. *Leuconostrum citrovorum* or *Pediococcus cerevisiae* is active only for folinic acid, which is sometimes referred to as citrovorum factor (5_N-formyl THF). Thus by differential microbiological assay one can make some distinction among the concentrations of circulating folates. While *L. casei* will respond to all forms of folate it will not distinguish the monoglutamates from the polyglutamates.

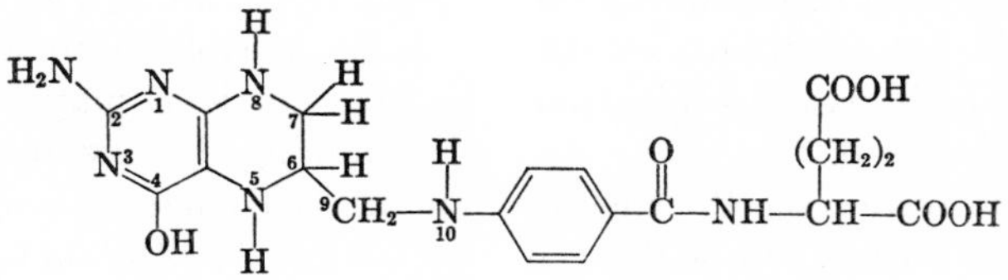

5,6,7,8 Tetrahydrofolic Acid

FIGURE 1

Pteroylpolyglutamates, the natural forms found in food, are presumably modified during absorption to yield mainly a reduced pteroylglutamate (THF). What is not entirely clear is where in the process of absorption the reduction actually occurs. Folates are most likely absorbed passively since their concentration in the normal diet far exceeds that in serum or blood. This reviewer believes that the present evidence strongly suggests that the major form of serum folate is the 5_N-methyl THF (V. Herbert, A. R. Larrabee, and J. M. Buchanan, *J. Clin. Invest.* **41**, *1134* (*1962*)). The table lists the various organisms used to assay folate activity and the forms for which they are active. *Lactobacillus casei* responds to essentially all forms of folate, while *Streptococcus faecalis* is apparently active only for the monoglutamate either in

The form folate takes in the red cell may be different from that found in the liver, serum, or other tissues. Evidence has been presented that the folate form in red cells is predominantly a polyglutamate or conjugated derivatives of 5_N-methyl THF; treatment of red cells with a conjugase prepared from chicken livers increases folate levels active for *L. casei* alone.

There are five known coenzyme forms of folacin, and their major role is in the transfer of one-carbon units to appropriate metabolites in the synthesis of DNA, RNA, methionine, and serine (A. L. Luhby and J. M. Cooperman, *Advances in Metabolic Disorders* **1**, *263* (*1964*)). Perhaps the two reactions which contribute most to the one-carbon pool are those involving conversion of serine to glycine, and of histidine to glutamic acid. In the serine to glycine re-

PGA--------Reduced--------THF

	Mono-Gluta-mate	Natural Poly-Gluta-mate		Mono-Gluta-mate	Natural Poly-Gluta-mate	5_N-methyl	"Normal" Serum Folate (ng/ml)
L. casei:	+	+		+	+	+	5–17
S. faecalis:	+	–		+	–	–	0– 2
P. cerevisiae:	–	–		+	–	–	0– 2

TABLE 1

action, THF is methylated to 5_N—10_N methylene THF (5_N—CH_2—10_N); this form being essential for DNA synthesis. Form-iminoglutamic acid (FIGLU), an interme-diate in the conversion of histidine to glu-tamic acid, loses its formimino group (—CH=NH) to THF, resulting in the formation of glutamic acid and 5_N— formimino THF. In folate deficiency or impaired utilization, urinary FIGLU is increased.

Another coenzyme form, 5_N—10_N methe-nyl THF (—5_N=CH—10_N), can be derived either from formimino THF or 5_N—10_N methylene THF. Formate arising from the metabolism of choline to glycine or from tryptophan reacts with THF to form still another coenzyme form, 10_N—formyl THF (10_N—CH=O). In the biosynthesis of me-thionine, 5_N—methyl THF is the coenzyme form, and in this reaction, which appears to require vitamin B_{12} as a cofactor, the methyl group is used to methylate homocys-teine, forming methionine. THF is thus regenerated in this reaction and is now available to "pick up" additional one-carbon units for synthesis of DNA and RNA.

The preponderance of evidence suggests that folate deficiency is extremely difficult to produce in mammals unless a folic acid antagonist is administered, or a vitamin C deficiency is induced, or unless iodinated casein, intestinal germicidal substances, or a high level of methionine is added to a diet already deficient in folic acid (G. M.

Briggs, *Am. J. Clin. Nutrition* **7**, *390* (*1959*)). Dietary folic acid deficiency may be equally difficult to produce in man. Perhaps it is worthwhile to stress at this point that administration of a nutrient to an ill patient, at whatever dose, which causes remission of a sign(s) or symptom(s) usually attributed to a dietary deficiency of that nutrient, may be of little value in determining dietary requirements for nor-mal man. To determine folacin requirements for normal, healthy man, Herbert (*Tr. Assn. Am. Phys.* **75**, *307* (*1962*)) placed himself on a low folate diet (less than 5 µg. of "folate" per day) and reported that after four months on such a regimen he developed megaloblastic anemia, at present a *sine qua non* sign of folate or vitamin B_{12} deficiency.

From this and other studies (R. Zalusky and Herbert, *New Engl. J. Med.* **265**, *1033* (*1961*)) the conclusion was drawn that the dietary requirement for folate was in the order of 50 µg. per day. H. Velez, A. Re-strepo, J. J. Vitale, and E. E. Hellerstein (*Am. J. Clin. Nutrition* **19**, *27* (*1966*)) fed low folate diets (less than 8 µg. per day) to six patients who had severe iron de-ficiency anemia due to hookworm infesta-tion and who had megaloblastic marrow maturation. The six patients recovered with iron therapy; all were discharged in three to four months with normoblastic marrows. G. Goldsmith (Personal Com-munication) also fed low folate diets to four patients, one for a period of up to eight months, and none of these developed any sign of folate deficiency despite serum folate levels of 1 ng. per milliliter or lower.

Thus the serum folate level may not be predictive of folate deficiency. Indeed, there is still some question as to whether man, like the rat, may not derive enough folate from bacterial synthesis (intestinal flora) to meet daily requirements. Further, FIGLU may also be of little value in diagnosing dietary folate deficiency, since this compound is found in excess amounts after histidine loading in patients with vitamin B_{12} deficiency, neoplastic disease, thyrotoxicosis, or iron deficiency.

In sprue, or in other diarrheal and malabsorption states, megaloblastic anemia may be a concomitant finding. T. W. Sheehy et al. (Blood **18**, 623 (1961)) demonstrated that 25 μg. of PGA per day effected a remission of the megaloblastosis in a high percentage of patients who were already ingesting approximately 1,000 to 1,300 μg. of dietary folate. It was postulated that such patients may have a defect in the production and/or secretion of enzyme(s) necessary for splitting off glutamic acid residues from the dietary polyglutamates of folacin. H. Baker, O. Frank, and H. Sobotka (J. Am. Med. Assn. **187**, 119 (1964)) presented evidence that patients with nontropical sprue may lack these enzymes, which either conjugate folacin or deconjugate the polyglutamates to a form more readily absorbed; these authors found that pteroyltriglutamate was absorbed better than folacin or pteroyldiglutamate.

Another possible explanation of folate deficiency in malabsorption syndromes may be related to the entero-hepatic circulation of folacin. Baker, S. Kumar, and S. P. Swaminathan (Lancet **1**, 685 (1965)) studied excretion of folic acid in the bile of eight fasting persons, and in all cases folate activity of the duodenal fluid was higher than that of serum. Thus the sprue patient may deplete himself of body folate by in-efficient reabsorption of folate secreted into the gastrointestinal tract.

There are still other disease entities in which folate metabolism may be altered. The megaloblastic anemia seen in alcoholics has usually been attributed to poor dietary habits and low folate intakes. Recently, however, L. W. Sullivan and Herbert (J. Clin. Invest. **43**, 2048 (1964)) studied alcoholic patients with low serum folate levels and with megaloblastosis. The three patients were subsequently treated with folacin, but if these patients were given whiskey the bone marrow again became megaloblastic although the serum folate level apparently had been raised to normal values by administration of PGA. However, the effect of alcohol could be reversed by giving large amounts of folate. The mechanism by which ethanol may produce megaloblastosis is not clear, but the effect may be mediated through aberrations in the enzyme system(s) concerned with folate metabolism or one-carbon transfer.

In certain malignant syndromes, megaloblastosis may also be present. It has been argued that in such situations, where there is profound cell proliferation, there may be an "increased need" for folacin, but this theory has been questioned by some investigators. Anticonvulsant drugs have also been shown to produce megaloblastosis, and presumably such drugs act as anti-folic analogues.

Iron deficiency may also result in a functional defect in folate utilization. Vitale et al. (J. Nutrition **88**, 315 (1966)) showed that the activity of the enzyme formimino-transferase was significantly reduced in iron deficient animals and was associated with a marked increase in urinary excretion of FIGLU. Previously I. Chanarin, D. Rothman, and V. Berry (Brit. Med. J. **1**, 480 (1965)) demonstrated that adults with iron deficiency anemia also had abnormally increased urinary excretion of FIGLU after histidine loading. More recently Chanarin *et al.* (*loc. cit.*) concluded that the addition of iron to the diet of pregnant women reduced the frequency of megaloblastic anemia. They suggested that iron deficiency may "in the first instance produce folate deficiency" signs. Admittedly, their conclusion was not well supported by the data presented.

Still other studies have made reference to the link between iron deficiency and folate metabolism. In studies with iron deficient children, megaloblastic anemia or megaloblastic marrows are not always confined to cases with very low blood folic acid levels (Y. Matoth, R. Zamir, S. Bar-Shani, and N. Grassowicz, *Pediatrics* **33**, 694 (*1964*)). Rapid clearance of folate administered intravenously may be observed in uncomplicated iron deficiency anemia, although the rapid clearance may not necessarily infer folate deficiency but may instead indicate rapid utilization or "increased needs"; *e.g.*, pregnancy.

There is reasonably good evidence that in vitamin B_{12} deficient animals and human beings 5_N-methyl THF actually accumulates, and results in a relative deficiency of the THF necessary for transfer of one-carbon units for DNA and RNA synthesis. The results of several studies utilizing animals, bacteria, and human beings support the generally accepted view that vitamin B_{12} is an essential cofactor for the enzyme(s) system involved in the transfer of the methyl group of 5_N-methyl THF to homocysteine, and that in vitamin B_{12} deficiency serum and tissue 5_N-methyl THF "piles up." However, some believe that THF, and not 5_N—methyl THF, accumulates in vitamin B_{12} deficiency (human). They postulate that the increased urinary excretion of FIGLU in vitamin B_{12} deficient animals and human beings may be due to a defect in formimino-transferase, the enzyme involved in the transfer of the formimino group of FIGLU to THF. The authors fail to explain the observed effects of administered methionine in decreasing the urinary excretion of FIGLU in vitamin B_{12} deficient animals and man. The effect of methionine in mitigating many of the signs of vitamin B_{12} deficiency is thought to be related to its effect on the synthesis of 5_N—10_N methylene THF reductase, an enzyme involved in the conversion of 5_N—10_N methylene THF to the 5_N—methyl THF. This observation requires confirmation in mammals. In any case, inhibition of the folate reductase enzyme would be expected to prevent the "piling up" of 5_N—methyl THF in vitamin B_{12} deficiency.

Folacin deficiency, as distinguished from *dietary* folacin deficiency, from whatever cause appears to result in megaloblastic dysplasia, macrocytic anemia, and perhaps glossitis. It remains to be proved that folacin deficiency does in fact produce morphological changes in the gastrointestinal tract. Quite the contrary, morphological changes of the small bowel may precipitate folacin deficiency. Finally, it may well be that dietary folate deficiency is not a major problem; rather, secondary folate deficiency (induced folate deficiency) may be the more serious world health problem.

There is much to be learned about folate metabolism. Secondary folate deficiency may involve failure to absorb circulating entero-hepatic or dietary folate, increased urinary excretion of THF, increased destruction of folate, interference in the synthesis and/or activation of enzymes necessary for proper folate utilization, or the production of anti-folates. The mechanisms by which folate deficiency signs appear in neoplasia, thyrotoxicosis, iron deficiency, pregnancy, myeloproliferative diseases, and hemolytic processes are not entirely clear.

It would not have been possible to review all of the excellent papers which have appeared on the subject of folacin since the last "Present Knowledge" series published in 1956. The reader may find the references listed useful as well as the references contained therein.

CHAPTER XXVI

PRESENT KNOWLEDGE OF METHYL GROUPS IN NUTRITION

Wendell H. Griffith, Ph.D. and Helen M. Dyer, Ph.D.

Since the last review of methyl groups in nutrition appeared in the revised Present Knowledge volume in 1956, this review includes references only from 1955. In *Transmethylation and Methionine Biosynthesis* edited by S. K. Shapiro and F. Schlenk (*University of Chicago Press, 1965*) methyl compounds have been discussed relative to syntheses, to the pathways of metabolism, to intermediate metabolites, and to the enzymes and coenzymes involved in the reactions in microorganisms and mammalian tissues.

Labile methyl groups are both endogenous and exogenous in origin. The natural sources are largely limited to choline, betaine, and methionine. The biogenesis of choline appears to be universal in nature, and is the result of the transfer of three methyl groups to an acceptor which may be either free aminoethanol or phosphatidylaminoethanol.

The *de novo* neogenesis of labile methyl from a formate carbon in the organism requires folic acid. The folic acid-tetrafolic system provides a unique mechanism for reduction of carbon to a methyl group that can be transferred to a methyl acceptor. Choline is converted to betaine, and betaine to betaine aldehyde which, in turn, transfers one methyl group to tetrahydrofolic acid (THF). Cobalamin (vitamin B_{12}) plays a key role in the regulated transfer of the methyl group to THF. All three methyl groups of choline return to the one-carbon unit pool at the level of 10_N-hydroxymethyl-THF.

Information regarding the apoenzymes and coenzymes for each step is far from complete. Moreover, the extent to which the methylene group of $5_N,10_N$-methylene-THF can be transferred to acceptors by a reductive, methyl-forming process is unknown, and the question of the transmethylation of the methyl of 5_N-methyl-THF is poorly understood. A recent review discusses the role of folacin and its physiologically active form in methylation reactions, the relation to vitamin B_{12}, a possible cofactor, and the possible involvement of folic acid deficiency in a number of pathologic conditions (*Nutrition Reviews* **24,** *289* (*1966*)).

S-adenosylmethionine, called activated methionine, is the most important methyl donor to transmethylation reactions. It requires ATP for its synthesis from methionine in a reaction catalyzed by S-adenosylmethionine synthetase. Other transmethylations not involving activated methionine, and not requiring ATP, serve only for the synthesis of methionine.

Most nutrition studies concerning methyl groups utilize diets deficient in choline. Signs of a deficiency of labile methyl groups would be expected whenever the demands for choline phospholipids, or other methyl-containing metabolites, exceed the dietary supply of labile methyl groups and the capacity of the organism to carry out *de novo* synthesis. Thus, of equal importance with the choline content of the diets is the quantity and quality of protein (methionine and cystine contents) and the adequacy of folacin and cobalamin. The age of the animal and the species are also important. The effect is most critical in young, rapidly growing animals. A sharp increase in the choline dehydrogenase (oxidase) activity of the liver and kidneys has been reported to occur during the age period in which young rats are particularly susceptible to a lack of choline.

Fatty livers and kidney lesions continue to be of primary interest as manifestations of choline deficiency. Fat, accumulating in the center of the liver lobules, is due to hypolipotropism and in the periphery is said to be due to the activity of the anterior pituitary. In addition to the two classic manifestations of a choline deficiency, namely kidney damage and fatty livers, and the more recent interest in the possible role of choline in arteriosclerosis, choline deficiency has been associated with hemochromatosis and with liver cancer in rats.

The severe consequences of a lack of dietary choline have been described in such species as the rat, chick, turkey poult, and rabbit. Young guinea pigs grew poorly on choline deficient diets and died between the third and fourth weeks but only occasionally did animals show fatty infiltration of the liver (M. E. Reid, *J. Nutrition* **56,** *215* *(1955)*). Methionine, betaine, or ethanolamine would not serve individually as substitutes for choline, although a combination of methionine and monomethylaminoethanol permitted excellent growth. In guinea pigs fed a diet with choline for three weeks and then a choline free diet for three weeks, fat was beginning to accumulate in the liver (*see Nutrition Reviews* **15,** *339* *(1957)*).

Guinea pigs, like the chick and unlike the rat, were unable to methylate ethanolamine directly. Weanling male albino mice developed extremely fatty livers with a basal homocystine diet, with or without folacin and vitamin B_{12} (H. E. Sauberlich, *J. Nutrition* **68,** *141* *(1959)*). The presence of choline or betaine largely prevented the fat accumulation, and supplementing with choline, folacin, and B_{12} resulted in normal liver fat level.

Liver choline dehydrogenase activity was markedly reduced in mice fed the basal diet supplemented with homocystine alone. The reduction in enzyme activity was largely prevented by folacin and in part by B_{12}. Choline was effective but betaine was not. Unlike the rat and chick, the supplementation of methionine with choline, folacin, homocystine, and vitamin B_{12} in the diet of the mouse had relatively little effect (*see Nutrition Reviews* **18,** *58* *(1960)*). The requirement for choline in the baboon is lower than that in the rat (*Ibid.* **23,** *270* *(1965)*). A mild fatty liver developed in two months in the baboon, but did not progress during three additional months on the deficient diet. The lesion was reversible when choline was fed.

Investigations of the cause of the effect of protein in lipotropism suggested that in addition to methionine, amino acids such as threonine, lysine, and tryptophan may have specific effects unrelated to adequate protein for growth (*Nutrition Reviews* **14,** *278* *(1956)*). Whereas choline is implicated in transport of fat from the liver (as lecithin), and as necessary for fatty acid oxidation in the liver, threonine may have some specific action in fat oxidation.

Many choline deficient rats failed to survive temperatures of 1 to 3° C. for a six-week period (*see Nutrition Reviews* **14,** *284* *(1956)*). Less lipid was found in the kidneys and livers than in control choline deficient rats kept at 22° C. and death was attributed to other causes. Rats maintained in the cold with choline added to the diet showed a high incidence of fat deposition in the coronary arteries which was not seen in survivors without choline.

Omission of choline from the diet greatly influenced the difference in liver fat of rats fed vegetable and animal fats (*Ibid.* **15,** *219* *(1957)*). Long chain, saturated fatty acids caused deposition of greater amounts of fat than short chain, unsaturated fatty acids. It required 0.15 per cent choline chloride to reduce the level of liver fat resulting from 30 per cent butter fat in the diet compared with 0.12 per cent choline chloride with 30 per cent corn oil.

On low choline rations, with or without methionine and tryptophan supplements, liver fat was higher with butter fat than with corn oil but growth was better with butter fat. In a dose response study choline was three times as effective as betaine in preventing liver fat and renal lesions in growing, weanling rats fed a diet containing vitamin B_{12} and protein enough to maintain body weight without supplement (*Nutrition Reviews* **15,** *48 (1957)*). The effect of methionine was comparable to that of betaine at low levels on a molar basis, but it was progressively less effective at increasing concentrations. Normal liver fat was not obtained with methionine either with or without 0.2 per cent cystine.

A diet containing 16 per cent of unsaturated fatty acids and 3 per cent cholesterol appeared to be toxic to weanling rats (*Ibid.* **16,** *186 (1958)*). The symptoms resembled those of choline deficiency, and could be prevented if extra choline was included in the diet, or injected, or if fatty acids were given as triglycerides. The results illustrate the complex picture of fat absorption, transport, and excretion which can be obtained when all three processes are studied at the same time.

The failure to find elevated serum lipids in weanling rats fed 0.17 to 1.95 g. choline per 100 g. diet containing 40 per cent fat and 2 per cent cholesterol may be related to the resistance of rats to the development of atherosclerosis, and may be due to the efficient hepatic removal of blood lipids in this species (*Nutrition Reviews* **20,** *183 (1962)*). While there is essentially no difference in the fatty acid patterns of liver lipids in choline deficient and choline supplemented rats, the type of dietary fat and carbohydrate is an important determinant in the fatty acid composition of liver triglycerides, diglycerides, and phospholipids (*Ibid.* **23,** *189 (1965)*). It is of importance that the relationship between dietary fat and liver and depot lipid composition be illustrated, since alteration in the dietary fat patterns of man has been recommended as a means of lowering the serum cholesterol level and thereby preventing coronary heart disease.

The net synthesis of choline was approximately 7 mg. per 100 g. rat per day, or an amount equal to the preformed choline supplied by 10 g. of a diet containing 0.1 per cent choline (*Nutrition Reviews* **23,** *351 (1965)*). The turnover rates in the livers of rats were: phosphatidylserine, 442 minutes, phosphatidylethanolamine, 127 minutes, and phosphatidylcholine, 72 minutes. The rapid turnover of phosphatidylcholine, together with the rather limited synthesis, provides an adequate explanation of why choline becomes an essential nutrient under certain dietary conditions. In contrast to the increases with riboflavin and folic acid, a two-fold increase of choline in the diet of rats caused a significant decrease of total and free vitamin B_{12} in both livers and kidneys to approximately the level found with a very deficient diet (*Ibid.* **18,** *16 (1960)*). There was little or no change in hemoglobin level or in storage of choline in the liver and kidney.

In rats, choline is probably converted to carnitine or a carnitine derivative (*Nutrition Reviews* **18,** *52 (1960)*). Carnitine could not replace choline as a lipotropic factor in weanling rats. Carnitine with palmitate added to rat liver homogenates increased formation of ketone bodies but had no influence on carbon dioxide production. Results suggested that in female rats lecithin may be formed principally from methylation of phosphatidylethanolamine or phosphatidylserine and that synthesis of lecithin from diglyceride and cytidine diphosphocholine may be a more important pathway in the male (*Ibid.* **22,** *218 (1964)*).

Dermal fibrosis, necroses of tip of tail, of tips of digits, and of renal tubules, and lens opacity were induced in rats fed choline deficient diets with normal or high fat content when injected with 5-hydroxytryptamine (*Nutrition Reviews* **16**, *347* (*1958*)). The morphologic lesions may be the result of compression of small vessels of fat filled, tubular epithelial cells. Old rats showed no symptoms when fed a choline deficient diet, but symptoms developed when serotonin was given.

Methionine and other sources of labile methyl groups prolonged the survival of rats fed thyroactive material (iodinated casein) and casein as a source of protein (*Nutrition Reviews* **17**, *213* (*1959*)). Liver choline dehydrogenase activity was decreased in "hyperthyroid" rats fed casein as compared with those fed cooked pork.

The influence of intestinal bacteria in animal nutrition was implicated by the finding that 20 per cent sorbitol (a poorly digested carbohydrate), replacing a like amount of sucrose with a diet deficient in vitamins, prevented symptoms of the vitamin deficiency (*Nutrition Reviews* **18**, *182* (*1960*)). Enough choline appeared to have been synthesized in the intestine from sorbitol to prevent kidney damage but not enough to prevent fatty livers. 2-Amino-2-methyl-1-propane possesses anti-choline-like properties for the rat (*Ibid.* **15**, *277* (*1957*)). Larger amounts were required to produce kidney lesions in older than in younger rats, and the severity depended upon age.

The effect was overcome by choline supplements, but betaine, methionine, and casein had little effect. If choline is suddenly removed from the diet of older rats severe kidney lesions result. The effect of choline supplements has been investigated in rats with fatty livers produced by excess niacin in high fat diets (L. L. Rikans, D. Araka, and D. C. Ederquist, *J. Nutrition* **85**, *107* (*1965*)), and in fatty livers associated with ingestion of alcohol (W. S. Hartroft, E. A. Porta, and A. Suzuki, *Quart. J. Stud. Alcohol* **25**, *427* (*1964*)).

The experimental counterpart to human pigment cirrhosis has been produced in rats by feeding a choline deficient diet supplemented with extra iron (*Nutrition Reviews* **19**, *83* (*1961*)). The choline deficient diet without added ferric ammonium citrate produced fatty livers and cirrhosis but no hemochromatosis (*Ibid.* **23**, *189* (*1965*)).

Methylation and dehydroxylation of hydroxyaromatic compounds in the animal organism have attracted a great deal of study (*Nutrition Reviews* **15**, *311* (*1957*)), as have the formation and metabolism of physiologically active compounds by N- and O-methyltransferases (*Transmethylation and Methionine Biosynthesis, p. 71.;* F. L. Margolis, J. Roffi, and A. Jost; *Science* **154**, *275* (*1966*)).

As yet no direct association has been demonstrated with choline deficiency and any specific disease in man. However, choline is widely used to treat cirrhosis, hepatitis, and fatty livers.

Among other recent studies are those on: the effect of choline and sarcosine on mitochondrial dinucleotides (L. Szarkowska and M. Erecinska, *Acta Biochim. Polon.* **12**, *179* (*1965*)); the oxidation of choline in rat liver mitochondria (D. R. Wilken, T. Kagawa, and H. A. Lardy, *J. Biol. Chem.* **240**, *1843* (*1965*)); the effect of choline on hepatic ultrastructural changes associated with the intravenous administration of fat (N. W. King, L. D. Jones, H. Sasaki, and F. Schaffner, *Am. J. Clin. Nutrition* **16**, *88* (*1965*)); the chemical composition and enzyme content of plasma membranes isolated from rat liver (P. Emmelot, C. J. Bos, E. L. Benedetti, and P. H. Rümke, *Biochim. Biophys. Acta* **90**, *126* (*1964*)); serum and liver amylase and transaminase activities in choline-deficiency fatty liver and cirrhosis (S. J. Winawer, S. A. Broitman, L. S. Gottlieb, and N. Zamcheck, *Gastroenterology* **48**, *216* (*1965*)); muscular dystrophy and rabbits on a choline deficient diet (V. Srivastava, A. Devi, and N. K. Sarkar, *J. Nutrition* **86**, *298* (*1965*)); and many reports involving acetylcholine.

Chapter XXVII

PRESENT KNOWLEDGE OF COENZYME Q

Oswald A. Roels, Ph.D.

The coenzyme Q group of compounds was discovered independently by groups of workers in two widely different fields: one group was investigating the effects of vitamin A deficiency and the role of vitamin A in metabolism outside the visual cycle; the second group was studying the electron transport system in mitochondria.

The vitamin A workers discovered that a compound with an absorption maximum at 272 mμ. was present in much greater quantities in the unsaponifiable fraction of the livers of rats with a vitamin A deficiency than those of normal controls (J. S. Lowe, R. A. Morton, and R. G. Harrison, *Nature* **172,** *716* (*1953*)). The substance was extracted from the unsaponifiable fraction of vitamin A deficient rat liver and was called ubiquinone-50. Ubiquinone-50 was then isolated from pig heart, and the molecular structure of the compound was established (Morton *et al., Helv. Chim. Acta* **41,** *2343* (*1958*)). As these studies progressed, another group of workers was studying a possible role of lipids in mitochondrial electron transport systems, prompted by the discovery that alpha-tocopherol played a role in electron transport systems (A. Nason and I. R. Lehman, *Science* **122,** *19* (*1955*)). A systematic examination of the lipids extracted from such widely different sources as beef heart and cauliflower mitochondria showed that a product with a sharp ultraviolet absorption maximum at 275 mμ. could be found in these extracts. The compound with this 275 mμ. absorption maximum was isolated from beef heart mitochondria and called coenzyme Q-10 (F. L. Crane, Y. Hatefi, R. L. Lester, and C. Widmer, *Biochim. Biophys. Acta* **25,** *220* (*1957*)). K.

Folkers and his collaborators (D. E. Wolf *et al., J. Am. Chem. Soc.* **80,** *4752* (*1958*)) established that both substances were identical and had the following structure:

Coenzyme Q-10 = Ubiquinone-50

Both names, coenzyme Q and ubiquinone, have been utilized ever since the discovery of this series of compounds. The number following the ubiquinone nomenclature indicates the number of carbon atoms in the isoprenoid side chain, whereas the number following coenzyme Q indicates the number of isoprenoid groups in the side chain.

Soon after this work, homologs of ubiquinone-50 with 45, 40, 35, and 30 carbon atoms in the side chain were isolated from different microorganisms (Lester and Crane, *Biochim. Biophys. Acta* **32,** *492* (*1959*); V. Gloor *et al., Helv. Chim. Acta* **41,** *2357* (*1958*)).

Morton and his collaborators, who had been responsible for the discovery of ubiquinone-50 in vitamin A deficient rat liver, found that a second substance with an absorption maximum at 283 mμ. could also be isolated from the unsaponifiable fraction of vitamin A deficient rat liver. They soon found that the same substance was also in the normal human kidney. They then saponified about 100 pounds of human kidneys and extracted the unsaponifiable material; by chromatographic purification, they obtained 153 mg. of a crystalline product, which they called ubichromenol-50

(D. L. Laidman, Morton, J. Y. F. Paterson, and J. F. Pennock, *Chem. Ind., 1019 (1959)*; *Biochem. J.* **74,** *541 (1960)*). Ubichromenol-50 has the following structure:

Ubichromenol-50

Ubiquinone-50 can easily be converted to ubichromenol-50 *in vitro* by adsorbing ubiquinone-50 on alumina, followed by elution with acetone containing 10 per cent hydrochloric acid (J. Links, *Biochim. Biophys. Acta* **38,** *193 (1960)*). J. Green and collaborators (Green, E. E. Edwin, A. T. Diplock, and D. McHale, *Biochem. Biophys. Res. Commun.* **2,** *269 (1960)*), however, claimed that ubiquinone-50 was not converted to the corresponding chromenol when adsorbed on alumina columns. This controversy then gave rise to the question of whether ubichromenol was a naturally occurring compound in the tissues of animals or mainly an artifact produced in the course of isolation of the compound from unsaponifiable material. This controversy was clearly settled by F. W. Hemming, Morton, and Pennock (*Biochem. J.* **80,** *445 (1960)*), who demonstrated that the compound they had isolated from human kidney was ubichromenol-50 because it was optically active, whereas ubichromenol-50 prepared by the cyclization of ubiquinone-50 is racemic.

The coenzyme Q group of compounds is widely distributed. They are found in many different organisms, in soybeans, many vegetable oils, in protozoa, and in a wide variety of animal tissues.

A comprehensive review of the ubiquinone and the coenzyme Q group of compounds has been published by O. Wiss and Gloor (*Vitamins and Hormones* **18,** *485 (1960)*). The isolation, the structural determination, the synthesis, and the biosynthesis of the coenzyme Q group of compounds were discussed fully by A. F. Wagner and Folkers in *Vitamins and Coenzymes, p. 435 (John Wiley & Sons, Inc., New York, 1964)*. An excellent review of vitamins and ubiquinone status in animals has recently been published by Hemming and Pennock (*Biochemistry of Quinones, R. A. Morton, Editor, p. 287. Academic Press, New York, 1965*).

The isoprenoid side chain of ubiquinone is biosynthesized from acetate or mevalonate. R. E. Olson and co-workers have demonstrated that phenylalanine is the precursor of the benzoquinone ring of ubiquinone (*Biochem. Biophys. Res. Commun.* **5,** *443 (1961)*).

In carefully controlled studies, Morton and W. E. J. Phillips (*Biochem. J.* **73,** *416 (1959)*) demonstrated that both ubiquinone and ubichromenol increase in the liver of vitamin A deficient rats. It was found (Hemming, Pennock, and Morton, *Biochem. J.* **68,** *29P (1958)*) that this increase of ubiquinone in vitamin A deficient rat liver was mainly associated with the microsomal and supernatant fractions, whereas the concentration of this compound in the mitochondria remained about the same as that in the mitochondria of the liver from normal rats, where the bulk of the ubiquinone is associated with those subcellular particles. Vitamin A deficiency did not cause detectable changes in the ubiquinone level in the liver of chickens, whereas vitamin A deficiency either lowers or does not affect the liver ubiquinone level in the guinea pig. V. C. Joshi and T. Ramasarma (*Biochim. Biophys. Acta* **115,** *294 (1966)*) have recently demonstrated that the accumulation of ubiquinone in vitamin A deficient rat liver is probably due to impaired catabolism of the compound rather than to increased synthesis.

Many authors have studied the effect of vitamin E deficiency on tissue levels of ubiquinone in experimental animals. Although conflicting results have been reported, it would appear that vitamin E deficiency does not influence tissue ubiquinone levels in the rat. In rabbits, however, ubiquinone levels were lower in the heart, liver, skeletal muscle, and body fat of vitamin E deficient animals than in controls supplemented with tocopherol.

In view of the correlation between the vitamin A status of the animal and the ubiquinone level of its liver, Wiss, Gloor, and F. Weber (*Ciba Foundation Symposium "Quinones in Electron Transport," G. E. W. Wolstenholme and C. M. O'Connor, Editors. Little, Brown and Company, Boston, 1961*) undertook a study of the effect of dietary ubiquinone on chickens. They found that when ubiquinone was fed at the level of 8 mg. per kilogram of diet a very slight growth stimulation occurred in the chicks. However, in view of its wide distribution and synthesis by a wide variety of living organisms, ubiquinone is obviously not a dietary essential.

The metabolic function of coenzyme Q is apparently associated with the oxidation of succinate and reduced nicotinamide adenine dinucleotide; it appears to be involved in electron transport systems and may be an integral component of liver aldehyde oxidase (K. V. Rajagopalan, I. Fridovich, and P. Handler, *J. Biol. Chem.* **237**, *922* (*1962*)). B. T. Storey (*Arch. Biochem. Biophys.* **114**, *431* (*1966*)) has demonstrated that ubiquinone can be extracted with hexane-methanol-triethanolamine from beef heart electron transport particles.

Because of the structural similarity between the tocopherols and the members of the coenzyme Q group of compounds, the effect of dietary supplements of ubiquinone and its analogs on vitamin E deficiency was studied in different animals. E. Søndergaard, M. L. Scott, and H. Dam (*J. Nutrition* **78**, *15* (*1962*)) found that the onset of encephalomalacia and the beginning of muscular dystrophy could be delayed in chicks fed a vitamin E deficient diet if they were supplemented with ubichromenol or

with phytyl ubichromenol (*i.e.*, the chromenol with the same saturated side chain as the tocopherols). Ubiquinone-30 or ubiquinone-50 had no effect. The administration of alpha-tocopherol, however, was very much more efficient than that of ubichromenol in curing or preventing encephalomalacia and muscular dystrophy in the chick caused by a vitamin E deficient diet. The chromanol of hexahydrocoenzyme Q-4 prevented encephalomalacia in the vitamin E deficient chick; it also prevented the resorption-gestation syndrome in the vitamin E deficient rat and cured nutritional muscular dystrophy in the vitamin E deficient rabbit (J. L. Smith *et al.*, *Arch. Biochem. Biophys.* **101**, *388* (*1963*)). The chromanol of hexahydrocoenzyme Q-4 has the following structure:

Chromanol of hexahydro-coenzyme Q-4.

As far as is known, the chromanols of coenzyme Q do not occur naturally; they can be synthesized in the laboratory. The same chromanol of hexahydrocoenzyme Q-4 cured the vitamin E deficient *Rhesus* monkey of anemia and muscular dystrophy within a few days after its administration (J. S. Dinning, C. D. Fitch, C. H. Shunk, and Folkers, *J. Am. Chem. Soc.* **84**, *2007* (*1962*)). The same authors observed that anemic and dystrophic monkeys develop reticulocytosis on treatment with a normally synthesized body component, coenzyme Q_{10}. Complete remission of the anemia is effected by hexahydrocoenzyme Q_4 therapy (Fitch *et al.*, *Arch. Biochem. Biophys.* **112**, *488* (*1965*)). Fitch and Folkers (*Biochem. Biophys. Res. Commun.* **26**, *128* (*1967*)) found that hexahydrocoenzyme Q_4

and the 6-chromanol of hexahydrocoenzyme Q_4 protect erythrocytes of premature infants from hemolysis by H_2O_2.

Ubichromenol has been shown to have definite antioxidant properties *in vitro* (J. Bieri, in *Nutrition Reviews* **21,** *129, (1963)*). It has therefore been proposed that the vitamin E-like effect of some of the members of the coenzyme Q group of compounds may be related to their antioxidant properties. The very striking curative effect of the chromanol of hexahydro-coenzyme Q-4 on a wide variety of symptoms caused by vitamin E deficiency in the chick, the rat, the rabbit, and the *Rhesus* monkey should greatly stimulate further research in this field of lipid metabolism to establish the exact function of "vitamin E" and of the coenzyme Q group of compounds in metabolism at the cellular level. A broad statement declaring the "antioxidant properties" of these compounds is far from adequate to explain their function in metabolic reactions.

Chapter XXVIII

PRESENT KNOWLEDGE OF THE MINERALS

Harold H. Sandstead, M.D.

The development of rapid and sensitive spectroscopic methods of assay and the application of radioisotopic tracer techniques have made possible a "mushrooming" of knowledge of the role of minerals in the vital functions of the body. It has become increasingly evident that, though trace elements are ubiquitous in nature, deficiencies in man, as well as animals, may occur in the proper ecological setting.

The toxic effects of excess essential and nonessential minerals have been further clarified in the last ten years. H. A. Schroeder and J. J. Balassi (*J. Chronic Dis.* **14,** *236, 408* (*1961*)) have reviewed the cardiovascular-renal toxicity and effects on longevity of cadmium and lead in man and animals.

The animal body requires seven elements in macro amounts: calcium, chloride, magnesium, potassium, phosphorus, sodium, and sulfur; and at least seven in "trace" amounts: cobalt, copper, iodine, iron, manganese, selenium, and zinc. In addition, chromium, fluorine, and molybdenum appear to have an important role in human metabolism. Other trace elements found in significant amounts in man are reviewed by E. J. Underwood (*Trace Elements in Human and Animal Nutrition, Second Edition. Academic Press, New York, 1962*). They are probably important in human nutrition; however, their role is not yet established. A detailed review of the body chemical composition has recently been published by E. M. Widdowson and J. W. T. Dickerson (*Mineral Metabolism, vol. II A, C. L. Comar and F. Bronner, Editors, p. 1. Academic Press, New York, 1964*). The daily requirement of many of the elements is not known.

Sodium, potassium, chlorine, sulfur, iodine, manganese, molybdenum, chromium, and cobalt will be discussed in this chapter. Calcium, copper, magnesium, phosphorus, selenium, fluorine, zinc, iron, and cadmium are presented separately.

Sodium

In mammalian tissues sodium is involved in maintenance of osmotic equilibrium and body fluid pH and helps to transmit the nerve impulse. Through the agency of an energy dependent "pump" sodium is removed from the intracellular to the extracellular environment. This distribution is essential for normal cellular metabolism. The effect of severe malnutrition on the function of the "pump" and the metabolic consequences have been reviewed by J. Metcoff *et al.* (*Medicine* **45,** *331* (*1966*)). Severe sodium deprivation ultimately results in growth failure and death.

The requirement for sodium is determined by needs for growth, losses due to sweating and other body secretions, and the potassium content of the diet. The estimated average sodium intake in the United States is 3 to 7 g. (7.5 to 18 g. of table salt) per person (*Recommended Dietary Allowances, Sixth Edition. NAS-NRC publication 1146, Washington D.C., 1964*). An intake of 1 g. salt for each liter of water lost in excess of 4 liters has been suggested. However, it has been shown that an acclimatized individual may lose only 0.5 g. per liter, whereas an unacclimatized person loses 2 to 3 g. per liter of sweat. Adults tolerate an intake of 2 to 4 mEq per day for long periods, provided there are no abnormal losses.

Sodium is rapidly absorbed from the

stomach and small intestine. Parenteral administration in combination with other electrolytes and sugar is a useful therapeutic technique now widely applied in a variety of surgical and medical diseases.

The major organ of excretion and conservation is the kidney. Roughly 99.5 per cent of sodium filtered by the glomerulus is reabsorbed. Conservation is a complex event, controlled in part by the renin, angiotensin, aldosterone system, in response to plasma volume and effective arterial perfusion of the juxtaglomerular apparatus (J. O. Davis, C. C. J. Carpenter, and C. R. Ayers, *Circulation Res.* **11**, *171* (*1962*); J. J. Brown, D. L. Davis, A. F. Lever, and J. I. S. Robertson, *Lancet* **2**, *278* (*1963*)). In addition to the aldosterone mediated distal tubular sodium reabsorption, there is an incompletely understood proximal tubular mechanism, which appears to be influenced by the volume of extracellular fluid (F. C. Rector, Jr., G. Van Giesen, F. Kiil, and D. W. Seldin, *J. Clin. Invest.* **43**, *341* (*1964*)).

Aldosterone also increases conservation by the sweat and salivary glands, and increases intestinal absorption of the cation. Bone does not appear to play a large role in maintaining sodium homeostasis.

Hyponatremia is frequently encountered by the clinician. The significance of this finding is dependent on the disease, state of hydration, dietary intake of sodium, and previous use of diuretic agents. The complex interplay of these factors has been the subject of an extensive review by R. E. Fuisz (*Medicine* **42**, *149* (*1963*)).

The effect of chronic excess dietary sodium on cardiovascular function and the evolution of hypertension has received considerable attention (D. M. Hilkner, N. S. Wenkam, and I. J. Lichton, *J. Nutrition* **87**, *371* (*1965*)). It has been suggested that excessive salt ingestion by infants on a Western diet may play a part in the evolution of hypertension in adults. In view of this, a report documenting the large

amounts of sodium (40 to 60 mEq per day) in infant diets in the United States is of interest (*Nutrition Reviews* **25**, *82* (*1967*)). In the rat, excess dietary sodium will produce hypertension associated with degenerative vascular disease affecting arterioles and glomeruli. Increased dietary potassium has a protective effect (G. R. Meneely, J. Lemley-Stone, and W. J. Darby, *Am. J. Cardiol* **8**, *527* (*1961*)). Susceptibility to "salt hypertension" is in part genetically determined. Certain strains of rats are highly resistant.

The effects of chronic excess salt in man are less well defined. In support of the hypothesis that excess salt ingestion is a factor in the etiology of human hypertension is the finding of L. K. Dahl, M. G. Smilay, L. Silver, and S. Spraragen (*Circulation Res.* **10**, *313* (*1962*)) that hypertensive patients have a prolonged biological half life of sodium-22, suggesting the presence of a larger body sodium pool. Acute salt poisoning in infants has been reported by L. Finberg and C. N. Luttrell (*J. Am. Med. Assn.* **184**, *187* (*1963*)).

Dietary sodium restriction is a cornerstone in treatment of hypertension and congestive failure. Successful use of low salt diets requires education of the patient. Several publications are available for this purpose (*Sodium Restricted Diets: The Rationale, Complications and Practical Aspects of Their Use. NAS-NRC publication 325, Washington, 1954;* American Heart Association Booklets, *Strict Sodium Restriction, EM 58; Moderate Sodium Restriction, EM 58A,* and *Mild Sodium Restriction; EM 58B, American Heart Association, New York, 1960*).

Potassium

Potassium is primarily an intracellular cation. Its location is maintained by an energy-requiring mechanism related to the sodium pump. In this location the cation is, in large part, bound to protein, influences osmotic equilibrium, is in part responsible for resting transmembrane potential, and facilitates a number of enzyme reactions, including phosphorylation of creatine and those involving pyruvate kinase. It participates in uptake of neutral amino acids by cells (T. R. Riggs, L. M. Walker, and H. N. Christensen, *J. Biol. Chem.* **233,** *1479* (*1958*)) and influences carbohydrate metabolism in the intact animal. Prolonged potassium deprivation in the rat results in hypertrophy of the adrenal glands, postprandial hyperglycemia, and depletion of tissue glycogen stores. Uptake of glucose by cells is associated with a shift of extracellular potassium into the cell with the glucose.

The major excretory pathway is the kidney. In the absence of disease the body efficiently conserves the cation; dietary deficiency is, therefore, unlikely. Potassium depletion may be a significant complication of diarrhea, vomiting, diuretic administration, hyperaldosteronism, renal tubular defects, chronic lung disease with alkalosis, diabetic acidosis, and severe protein-colorie malnutrition. Rapidity of depletion and the ratio of intracellular to extracellular potassium, in part, determine the signs and symptoms.

For example, the ECG patterns in diabetic acidosis may be consistent with hyperkalemia even though there is serum hypokalemia and total body deficit in potassium. The therapeutic implications have been discussed by K. H. Stenzel, J. C. Dougherty, L. Sherr, and G. D. Lubash (*J. Am. Med. Assn.* **187,** *372* (*1964*)). Potassium depletion in patients with cirrhosis of the liver is not uncommon. A complication of the deficiency may be precipitation of hepatic coma, presumably due to increased renal ammonia production (G. J. Gabuzda and P. W. Hall, *Medicine* **45,** *481* (*1966*)).

Another complication of potassium deficiency in the rat is increased susceptibility to renal infection. Experimental infection can be produced before histologic lesions of deficiency appear (R. C. Muehreke and J. C. McMillan, *Ann. Int. Med.* **59,** *427* (*1963*)). Increased ammonia production by the potassium deficient kidney and alkalinity of the renal pyramids may account for this.

In man, if sodium is also restricted, potassium deficiency results in sodium retention, mild alkalosis, and mild hypokalemia. Alkalosis and hypokalemia are more severe if dietary sodium is increased. Correction of the alkalosis requires repletion of associated chloride deficits. This may be accomplished with sodium chloride in spite of continued potassium deficiency. Potassium conservation by the renal tubule appears to require the presence of chloride; for this reason potassium chloride is more effective than alkaline salts of potassium in repletion of potassium deficiency (J. de Graeff, A. Struyvenberg, and L. D. F. Lameijer, *Am. J. Med.* **37,** *778* (*1964*); J. P. Kassiver and W. B. Schwartz, *Ibid.* **40,** *19* (*1966*)).

Potassium and magnesium are intimately related in metabolism. Magnesium deficiency in the rat leads to a failure to retain potassium, and similar observations have been made in man (I. MacIntyre, S. Hanna, C. C. Booth, and A. E. Read, *Clin. Sci.* **20,** *297* (*1961*); V. P. Petersen, *Acta Med. Scandinav.* **174,** *595* (*1963*)).

Chronic potassium excess produces hypertrophy of the zona glomerulosa of the rat adrenal without affecting granulation of the juxtaglomerular apparatus. A form of secondary aldosteronism independent of the renin, angiotensin system is thereby produced (P. M. Hartroft and E. Sowa, *J. Nutrition* **82,** *439* (*1964*)).

In man, potassium excess is seldom a problem except in renal failure or severe acidosis. Hyperkalemia may be treated by potassium restriction, removal of potassium by gastrointestinal sodium exchange resins, correction of acidosis, and administration of glucose and insulin. Occasionally, extracorporeal hemodialysis is necessary.

For further consideration of potassium in

clinical medicine the reader is referred to B. H. Scribner and J. M. Burnell (*Metabolism* **5**, *468* (*1955*)) and D. C. Darrow and S. Helleistein (*Physiol. Rev.* **38**, *114* (*1958*)).

Chlorine

Nearly all dietary chlorine occurs as sodium chloride. Deficiency, therefore, occurs under the same circumstances as deficiency of sodium.

About two-thirds of blood anions are chlorine, 88 per cent being extracellular. Cerebral spinal fluid contains the highest concentration, followed by interstitial fluid, lymph, serous transudates, exudates, and gastrointestinal secretions. Extracellular chlorine is for all practical purposes a free anion, having a binding affinity for serum albumin one-fourth that of iodine and one-twentieth that of thiocyanate. Preservation of the extracellular location appears to be mediated by an active transport system; however, the physiologic purpose of maintenance of intracellular concentrations of 1 mEq per liter or less (rat muscle) is not known.

An important function of chlorine in the body is to act as a buffer. The contribution of erythrocyte chlorine to total buffering is in the range of 5 per cent in metabolic alkalosis, 10 per cent in metabolic acidosis, 30 per cent in respiratory acidosis, and 40 per cent in respiratory alkalosis.

Homeostasis of chlorine and homeostasis of potassium are intimately related: a deficiency of one will lead to a deficiency of the other.

Sulfur

Sulfur is an essential nutrient for both animals and plants. Plants utilize inorganic sulfate to synthesize organic sulfur compounds which animals consume. Higher animals require the presence of only three of these compounds in the diet: methionine, thiamine, and biotin. Usually the major source of sulfur in the human diet is cysteine. Much of this sulfur is utilized to synthesize sulphomucopolysaccharides. Other compounds containing sulfur include cystine, glutathione, coenzyme A, lipoic acid, and taurine. The various sulfa drugs, penicillin, and thiouracil are examples of pharmacologic agents containing sulfur.

Inorganic sulfur is poorly absorbed. Until recently it was thought unimportant in nutrition of higher animals. Using calcium sulfate and methionine labeled with sulfur-35, F. G. Michels and J. T. Smith (*J. Nutrition* **87**, *217* (*1965*)) have shown that inorganic sulfur is important in the diet of the rat. Inorganic sulfate contributes to the body's sulfate pool as does sulfur from organic compounds. Availability of sulfate for absorption is related to the ratio of organic to inorganic sulfur. Methionine absorption is influenced by the level of dietary inorganic sulfate.

The functions of compounds containing sulfur in the body are numerous. In connective tissue, decreased dietary sulfate impedes the collagen producing activity of fibroblasts, and *in vitro* gel formation by soluble collagen solutions (R. G. Brown, G. M. Button, and J. T. Smith, *J. Nutrition* **87**, *228* (*1965*)). Chondroitin sulfates are the sulphomucopolysaccharides affected.

Chondroitin sulfates appear to be synthesized in cartilage shortly before ossification (D. D. Dziewiatkowski, F. Bronner, N. DiFerrante, and G. Okinaka, *J. Exp. Med.* **106**, *509* (*1957*)). Synthesis may, in part, be influenced by a non-pituitary hormone: sulfation factor. The role of sulfation factor in growth regulation is currently under investigation (W. D. Salmon, Jr., *J. Lab. Clin. Med.* **56**, *673* (*1960*)). Severe malnutrition and deficiencies of vitamins A and C, growth hormone, and thyroxine impair chondroitin sulfate synthesis. Congenital abnormalities affecting connective tissue metabolism, such as Hurler's and Morquio's syndromes (V. A. McKusick *et al.*, *Medicine* **44**, *445* (*1965*)), result in urinary excretion of sulphomucopolysaccharides.

Other sulfated polysaccharides include the mucoitin sulfates and heparin. The former appear to function as gut lubricants. Heparin is synthesized by mast cells, inhibits coagulation, and on injection will induce appearance of a lipid clearing factor in the plasma.

Cysteine, cystine, methionine, and taurine are probably the most extensively studied compounds containing sulfur. Methionine will replace cysteine and cystine in the diet. It plays a central role in methyl transfer.

Cystine appears to have a specific function in muscle metabolism which cannot be substituted by methionine. M. L. Scott and C. C. Calvert (*Abstracts of the Fifth International Congress of Nutrition*, p. 77. *Washington, D.C., 1960*) found that cystine added to a diet deficient in vitamin E and low in methionine and cystine would prevent muscular dystrophy in chicks, whereas methionine would not.

Iodine

Since 1850 it has been known that goiter and creatinism occur in regions where environmental iodine is meager. Numerous observers have documented the relationship between iodine lack and endemic goiter. Consequently, iodine enrichment of salt has become the accepted method of eliminating the disease. Although there is some disagreement, it appears that any level of enrichment between 1 in 10,000 and 1 in 100,000 will be effective, provided the iodine does not decrease in storage. The recommended daily intake to prevent goiter in adults is 100 to 150 μg.

Foods rich in iodine come from the sea. Seaweeds concentrate large amounts (700,000 μg. per cent) of the halogen and have been used since antiquity to treat goiter. Paradoxically, people ingesting large amounts of the weed may show endemic goiter due to iodine excess (H. Suzuki *et al.*, *Acta Endocrinologica* **50,** *161 (1965)*). Non-marine plant and animal products are not good dietary sources.

R. H. Follis, Jr. (*Am. J. Trop. Med. Hyg.* **13,** *137 (1964)*) found urinary iodine excretion a useful screening method in population surveys. Iodine excretions below 50 mg. per gram of urinary creatinine are thought to indicate an inadequate dietary intake and an increased incidence of goiter. This relationship is probably not so simple. Other environmental, dietary (goitrogens), and genetic factors no doubt play a role. This concept has been tested experimentally in the rat by L. Jirousek and D. I. R. Reisenaur (*Endokrinologie* **41,** *343* (*1961*); *Endocrinologia Experimentalis*, **1,** *271* (*1964*)). Thyroid enlargement was found dependent on the interplay of these three factors.

Studies in man showed that 93 per cent of children and 75 per cent of adults in a Mexican village had goiter. Dietary iodine intake of ten of the children ranged from 34 to 128 μg. per day with a modal intake of 55 μg. per day, a value similar to the modal iodine intake of non-goitrous individuals in an iodine rich area, Bethesda, Maryland (64 μg. per day). Mexican children showed a strong positive iodine balance and low urinary excretion in contrast to children from Bethesda.

In a Kentucky village where the goiter incidence is 33 per cent (W. T. London, D. A. Koutras, A. Pressman, and R. L. Vought, *J. Clin. Endocrinol.* **25,** *1091* (*1965*)) intake of iodine in goitrous and non-goitrous individuals was similar and in the range of non-goitrous individuals in Bethesda. Mean urinary iodine excretion of the goitrous individuals was not significantly different from the non-goitrous. Iodine excretions were greater than the lower normal quoted by Follis. Goitrous individuals showed an increased uptake of stable iodine without an increase in serum protein bound iodine, suggesting that trapped iodine was not converted to thyroid hormone. These studies indicate that, although iodine deficiency is the major cause of endemic goiter, other factors contribute.

Some of the many factors interfering with iodine uptake by the thyroid are reviewed by R. R. Grayson (*Am. J. Med.* **34,** *397 (1960)*). The exact mechanism whereby the thyroid accumulates iodine is not known. L. W. Cunningham (*Biochemistry* **3,** *1629 (1964)*) has suggested an active carrier mechanism in which sulfhydryl groups complex with iodine to form a sulfenyl iodide. This suggestion helps explain the antithyroid action of thiouracil and thiourea, as they have high reaction rates with sulfenyl iodide. By complexing with the sulfur these compounds may form disulfide and inactivate the carrier.

Iodine deficiency has been thought to contribute to a number of pathological conditions. A relationship to creatinism associated with endemic goiter is established; a relationship to sporadic creatinism, deaf mutism, and feeble-mindedness is not. The latter condition appears to be due to a genetically determined block in the organification of iodine (M. E. Morgans and W. R. Trotter, *Lancet* **1,** *607 (1958)*). There is presently no consensus on a possible relationship between endemic goiter and carcinoma of the thyroid. A relationship between thyrotoxicosis and endemic goiter is also not established. Postulated effects of iodine deficiency such as growth failure and retarded mental development are poorly studied.

Manganese

The role of manganese in human nutrition is poorly understood. A deficiency has not been recognized in man; the requirement has been established on the basis of animal studies.

Manifestations of experimental deficiency in the rat and other species include retardation of growth, structural and chemical anomalies of bone, ataxia, female sterility, male impotence, and abnormalities of lipid metabolism. As a result of suppression of epiphyseal cartilage cell proliferation, decreased matrix formation, and failure of endochondral bone growth, bowing of bones, fractures, joint deformities, and tendon slippage occur. Chondrodystrophy in chicks and perosis in older birds are striking examples of experimental deficiency and the importance of manganese in bone metabolism, where it apparently influences mucopolysaccharide synthesis.

Irreversible ataxia and seizure phenomena occur in newborn chicks, rats, guinea pigs, and swine from mothers deficient in manganese. Defects in structure of the vestibular apparatus occur. The seizures are thought due to uncharacterized metabolic abnormalities in the cerebral cortex. The relationship of these observations to the finding that manganese supplementation will prevent ataxia and loss of righting reflex in a strain of rats with this genetic abnormality is at present unclear (L. Hurley, L. Erway, and A. Fraser, *Fed. Proc.* **25,** *432 (1966)*).

Manganese deficiency results in infertility in a variety of species and poor milk production in swine and cattle. These manifestations may be related to incompletely understood interactions between choline and manganese and a lipotropic effect of manganese.

In vitro manganese with valence $+2$ activates many of the same enzymes as magnesium (*e.g.*, deoxyribonuclease, phosphatases, arginase, exopeptidases, dipeptidases, cysteine desulfhydrase). Application of this information to *in vivo* systems is perhaps unwarranted, as manganese *in vivo* has a valence of $+3$.

Absorption is increased in iron deficiency. This is thought to indicate that the mechanisms of manganese and iron absorption are similar (S. Pollack *et al.*, *J. Clin. Invest.* **44,** *1470 (1965)*). Absorbed manganese, valence $+2$, is oxidized to manganese, valence $+3$, and bound by a specific transport beta-1-globulin, transmanganin. Tissues rich in mitochondria concentrate and take up the metal. Its function appears to be specific and related to oxidative phosphorylation; intracellular and extracellular manganese are in dynamic equilibrium; other metals will not displace manganese from its intracellular location. The whole blood concentration of manganese by neutron activation is 2.4 ± 0.8 μg. per 100 ml., half of which is extracellular. Conservation is efficient. The major route of excretion is biliary, and most of what is excreted is reabsorbed.

Man's daily requirement of manganese is unknown. Factors thought to influence its absorption and retention include amount and availability in the diet, fat free body weight, and metabolic rate. A group of men on vegetarian diets was found to retain 0.04 mg. manganese per kilogram body weight from a diet containing 7.07 mg. (V. M. Lang, B. B. North, and L. M. Morse, *J. Nutrition* **85,** *132* (*1965*)). Nine-year-old children have been found to retain 0.05 mg. per kilogram body weight. Two-year-olds retained 0.2 mg. per kilogram from a diet providing 3.2 mg. per day (*Nutrition Reviews* **23,** *236* (*1965*)). The occidental diet contains roughly 4 mg. per day, an amount apparently adequate.

Foods particularly rich in manganese are the "genetic materials" of plants (seeds and nuts). Removal of outer layers of grains in milling results in loss of much of the manganese. Animal products are not rich sources.

Manganese intoxication in man (*e.g.* miners) is primarily an industrial hazard and is typically chronic. Manifestations include weakness, psychological disorders, and extrapyramidal, pyramidal, and cerebellar motor difficulties. Pathologic lesions occur in the basal ganglia, frontal lobes, and cerebellum. Treatment with chelating agents has met with varying success (S. A. El Naby and M. Hassanein, *J. Neurol., Neurosurg., Psychiat.* **28,** *282* (*1965*)).

Molybdenum

Man's requirement for molybdenum is inferred by the presence of the cation in xanthine oxidase and certain flavoproteins.

The amount required is probably minute, as it has been shown that rats fed as little as 0.2 μg. per day continue to grow, and that xanthine oxidase activity is retained. Deficiency symptoms and growth failure have been produced in the chick.

The interrelationship between molybdenum, copper, and sulfur in metabolism has received considerable attention. The molybdenum-copper relationship in nature was first observed in cattle, grazing on pastures rich in molybdenum. They developed signs and symptoms consistent with copper deficiency which respond to treatment with copper. Molybdenum and copper appear to compete for the same metabolic sites. As a result of excess molybdenum, blood and urine content of copper increase while bile and intestinal secretion of copper decrease. Concentrations of copper in renal and liver parenchyma increase. Cattle develop diarrhea, achromotrichia, brittle bones, and weight loss. Bone abnormalities are characterized by cartilagenous hyperplasia and diminished osteoblastic activity somewhat similar to osteolathyrism.

Adding sulfate to a diet high in molybdenum will prevent signs of intoxication, in part, by increasing molybdenum excretion. The amount of sulfate is important: excessive amounts will increase signs of toxicity.

Effects of excess copper on molybdenum metabolism are less well studied. It is known that nitrate reductase activity of *Neurospora crassa* is decreased, an effect opposed by molybdenum.

Trace metal deficiencies in plants are a possible etiologic factor in the occurrence of esophageal carcinoma in Bantu women of South Africa (R. J. W. Burrell, W. A. Roach, and A. Shadwell, *J. Nat. Cancer Inst.* **36,** *201* (*1966*)). Trace mineral deficiencies, molybdenum in particular, in corn and other plants allow certain fungi to grow on the plants. These fungi (*e.g., Aspergillus flavus*) produce mycotoxins carcinogenic for the rat. In addition, carcinogenic nitrosamines may accumulate in the molybdenum deficient plant. The extreme complexity of the ecology of nutritional disease is illustrated by this study.

Chromium

Prior to recent investigation of trivalent chromium's possible role in diabetes mellitus, the metabolic importance of chromium in man was unknown. In 1959, trivalent chromium was found to be necessary for normal glucose tolerance in the rat. Subsequent studies showed that minute amounts (0.1 μg.) increased the uptake of glucose by *in vitro* rat epididymal fat tissue by 90 per cent in the presence of 1 milliunit of insulin and that a non-utilizable sugar, D-galactose, behaved in a manner similar to glucose. In human diabetes mellitus, glucose tolerance improved in three of six patients following treatment with 180 to 3,000 μg. daily for 15 to 133 days. Normal individuals were unaffected. Other investigators have reported similar observations (*see Nutrition Reviews* **25,** *49* (*1967*)).

Deficiency of trivalent chromium apparently may occur in severe protein-calorie malnutrition. The impaired glucose utilization which occurs in kwashiorkor is temporarily corrected by oral administration of 250 μg. trivalent chromium. On the basis of these studies trivalent chromium appears to be a glucose tolerance factor for man as well as the rat. It is not a hypoglycemic agent, but increases the effectiveness of insulin, perhaps by forming a ternary complex between sulfhydryl groups of the insulin molecule and the cell membrane (*Nutrition Reviews, loc. cit.*).

The usual daily intake of chromium ranges from 30 to 80 μg.; very little is absorbed and retained. The daily requirement is unknown. It is distributed between the organs of the body in a fairly uniform manner, with approximately 0.02 to 0.64 p.p.m. in wet tissue. Beef liver nucleoprotein contains 1.80 p.p.m. In this location it has been thought to play a role in maintenance of the configuration of the ribonucleic acid molecule through formation of convalent bonds (W. E. C. Wacker and B. L. Vallee, *Fed. Proc.* **18,** *345* (*1959*)). Of interest is Tipton's (*Metal Binding in Medicine, M. J. Daven and L. A. Johnson, Editors, p. 27. Lippincott, Philadelphia, 1960*) finding that body chromium decreases with age. Perhaps this tendency may be in some way related to the increased incidence of diabetes and degenerative vascular disease in older people.

Cobalt

The need for cobalt in human nutrition appears to be entirely due to its presence in the vitamin B_{12} molecule. At present there is no evidence to suggest that this cation has any other function in human metabolism.

A cobalt cycle is present in nature. Cobalt is obtained from the soil by plants. Ruminants ingest the plants, and bacteria in the rumen utilize the cobalt to manufacture vitamin B_{12}. The animal absorbs the B_{12} and the vitamin is distributed throughout the body. Highest concentrations are found in liver (50 to 100 μg. per cent in beef liver), muscle contains 2 to 8 μg. per cent, and small but significant amounts are present in milk. Meat and animal products are ingested by man and other non-ruminants. A factor secreted by the gastric mucosa facilitates absorption of B_{12} (maximal in the ileum). Failure to produce intrinsic factor (pernicious anemia) and certain post-surgical and other gastrointestinal abnormalities (gastrectomy, resection of the ileum, blind loops, diverticulae) may interfere with absorption. The daily requirement of B_{12} is minute (approximately 1 μg. per day). Therefore, primary nutritional deficiency is extremely rare except in people who ingest no animal products.

Biochemical functions of B_{12} are incompletely understood. It plays a role in the metabolism of nucleic acids, carbohydrates, and fats. Discussion of these functions may be found in *Medicine* (**43,** *615* (*1964*)).

Cobalt has the same function in other animal species as in man. Ruminants may become deficient from grazing pastures in which cobalt is low. Monogastric animals (pigs, rats, chicks) maintained on a pure vegetable ration will develop B_{12} deficiency if coprophagy is prevented.

Cobalt salts in amounts of approximately 1 mg. per day per kilogram will induce polycythemia in many species. The mechanism of this phenomenon is unknown. Advantage has been taken of this erythropoietic stimulating effect in treating anemia due to uremia, infection, and sickle cell disease.

Side effects include goiter and hypothyroidism. E. Pimental-Malaussena, M. Roche, and M. Layrisse (*J. Am. Med. Assn.* **167,** *1719* (*1958*)) have used the antithyroid effect of cobalt in experimental treatment of thyrotoxicosis. Four of eight patients failed to respond to the drug. Use of cobalt salts in treating anemia is not without risk and should only be done, if at all, with careful follow-up.

It has been suggested that cobalt increases efficiency of iron utilization. This apparent action may be due to its polycythemic effect. Use of cobalt in treatment of iron deficiency is certainly not justified; the effect of cobalt salts being pharmacologic, the side effects significant, and the anemia responsive to iron alone.

CHAPTER XXIX

PRESENT KNOWLEDGE OF IRON AND COPPER

JAMES C. PEDEN, JR., M.D.

Iron is an element which is required for life. It is necessary for the production of hemoglobin, the myoglobin of muscles, and certain essential enzymes. The normal human adult body contains between 3 and 5 g. of iron—55 to 60 per cent in hemoglobin, 30 to 35 per cent in storage forms, and the remainder in various tissue components and enzymes.

Iron is held tenaciously by the body, and what is released in the process of hemoglobin breakdown re-enters the iron pool and is largely reutilized for more hemoglobin synthesis. Thus the body's need for iron is normally only for replacement of that small amount lost in the urine (less than 0.1 mg. per day), the feces (0.3 to 0.5 mg. per day), and the sweat, and by exfoliation of cells of the skin (in an amount which is still the subject of some controversy). The loss of iron by these mechanisms totals approximately 0.5 to 1.0 mg. per day.

Under certain normal circumstances, iron loss from the body is increased. In the menstruating female, an additional 0.3 to 1.0 mg. per day is required to compensate for the hemoglobin iron lost in menstrual blood. In pregnancy and childbirth, the "cost" in iron stores may range from 0 to 2 mg. per day for the duration of pregnancy and lactation. In growing children, iron needs are increased. The increase varies with age but averages about 0.6 mg. per day for the period from birth to the cessation of growth.

Iron requirements can thus be summarized: adult males and post-menopausal females, 0.5 to 1 mg. per day; menstruating females, 1 to 2 mg. per day; pregnant fe-

males, 1.5 to 2.5 mg. per day; children, on the average, 1 mg. per day; girls from 12 to 15 years of age, 1 to 2.5 mg. per day (C. V. Moore, in *Iron Metabolism, F. Gross, Editor, p. 251. Springer-Verlag, Berlin (1964)*). To these needs must be added iron required to replace that lost by any abnormal blood loss.

Ordinarily, these needs must be met by the iron content of the diet. Certain foods such as meat, particularly liver and kidneys, and green vegetables are rich in iron. However, the "availability" of iron for intestinal absorption varies considerably from one food to another and has been measured for only a few foods. It is generally true that absorption of iron from food sources is not as good as absorption from inorganic iron salts administered therapeutically. From the average diet probably 5 to 10 per cent of food iron is absorbed. This absorption is increased in the iron deficient subject, and may vary with alterations in the composition of the diet (*Nutrition Reviews* **22**, *306* (*1964*)). The percentage of iron absorbed from meat, liver, and enriched bread is greater than that absorbed from eggs or green vegetables (Moore, *loc. cit., p. 243*). An important source of iron in the diet, which is often overlooked, is the iron to be found in some water supplies, in wines and beers, and that which enters foodstuffs during cooking in iron vessels.

The actual iron content of the diet of different peoples is not precisely known. Most information that is available has been obtained from dietary surveys rather than by actual analysis of foods eaten. In the United States the iron content of the diet of the average city dweller has been estimated to be between 16 and 18 mg. per day. In other parts of the world and in lower income groups dietary iron content may be significantly less.

If it is assumed that 10 per cent of dietary iron is absorbed, it is clear that dietary sources of iron in the United States will be adequate for the postmenopausal female and the adult male and most children. It is also obvious that some menstruating females, pregnant women, and adolescent girls may require iron supplementation to maintain adequate body iron stores.

It has long been known that the ferrous salts of inorganic iron compounds are much more readily absorbed than the corresponding ferric salts. It has also been known that maximal absorption of iron occurs in the upper small intestine, and that the greater acidity of the intestinal contents at this level is of importance in keeping dietary iron available for absorption. In recent years, foods have been made available that have been grown or produced in an environment containing radioactively labeled iron salts, and absorption studies using tagged food iron in place of simple inorganic iron salts have yielded some surprising information. For instance, absorption of iron from enriched bread is no different whether ferrous sulfate or iron in the form of ferric orthphopshate or sodium ferric pyrophosphate is incorporated into the bread (R. Steinkamp, R. Dubach, and Moore, *Arch. Int. Med.* **95**, *181* (*1955*)).

The effect of gastric acid on food iron absorption is somewhat uncertain, since some workers report no effect of achlorhydria on the absorption of food iron, and others have presented contrary results. The number of individual foods studied with these techniques has been small, and clarification of the problems of absorption of food iron must await further studies.

Regulation of iron absorption in the intestine is a complicated matter which is not thoroughly resolved. It is known that cer-tain conditions and manipulations will markedly increase the percentage of iron absorbed from the diet. Ascorbic acid, when administered orally, increases absorption of iron from most foods. An increased rate of erythropoiesis in association with certain hemolytic anemias, hypoxia, and the like, will increase gastrointestinal absorption of iron. A reduction in the intestinal secretions of the pancreas, as by duct ligation, will increase iron absorption. Starvation, pregnancy, pyridoxine deficiency, and other miscellaneous conditions are also associated with increased iron absorption. Most importantly, depletion of the body's iron stores results in an increased percentage absorption of iron from the diet.

Until recently, control of iron absorption had been explained by the "mucosal block" theory proposed some years ago (S. Granick, *Science* **103**, *107* (*1946*)). According to this theory iron absorption was mediated obligatorily by an iron-accepting protein of the intestinal cell. This protein is apoferritin. The apoferritin-iron complex is ferritin. Iron absorption was thus limited under normal circumstances by the availability of apoferritin in the mucosal cell. It was postulated that, in times of increased iron need, the oxidizing potential at the mucosal border of the luminal cells is lost, allowing ferrous iron to diffuse directly across the cell and into the plasma without mediation of the apoferritin-ferritin system.

Certain recent experimental results have caused objections to be raised to the "mucosal block" theory. It has been noted, most importantly, that some small percentage of orally administered iron continues to be absorbed in spite of preloading of the body with large quanities of iron given either orally or systemically. It has been shown also that in absolute terms, absorption of iron increases with increasing oral dosages which are limited only by the toxicity of iron. It has not been possible experimentally to demonstrate measurable differences in oxidation-reduction potentials at the luminal and vascular borders of the intestinal cell.

For these reasons and others it is now felt that iron from the intestinal lumen enters the mucosal cells either in an ionic form or bound to a low molecular weight non-protein substance. This entrance of iron is not felt to be an energy requiring process. In the cell, the iron complex diffuses directly to the vascular border, where the iron is transferred across the cell membrane into the plasma by a process that does require oxidative energy and appears to be the rate limiting reaction (E. B. Dowdle, D. Schachter, and H. Schenker, *Am. J. Physiol.* **198,** *609 (1960)*). Iron that is not rapidly transported into the plasma is thought to accumulate in the cell and complexes with apoferritin to form ferritin. In this system the apoferritin and ferritin are no longer considered obligatory intermediates in normal iron absorption.

Iron is transported in the plasma bound to a protein which has been called transferrin or siderophilin. The protein is formed in the liver and is normally present in the plasma in a concentration sufficient to bind 280 to 400 μg. of iron per 100 ml. of plasma. This iron binding capacity of the plasma is increased in iron deficiency, in pregnancy, and in hypoxic states, and is decreased in association with certain inflammatory reactions and infections, and may be decreased in states of severe protein malnutrition.

Iron is cleared from the plasma with a half time of 60 to 120 minutes either into the erythroid precursors of the bone marrow or into storage complexes. Total iron turnover in the body is of the order of 25 to 40 mg. per day. The plasma iron clearance rate is increased in iron deficiency and when erythropoiesis is accelerated. It is reduced in the face of erythroid hypoplasia of the bone marrow. Under circumstances of normal erythropoietic activity up to 90 per cent of iron absorbed and passing through the plasma compartment will enter the

bone marrow and some 70 per cent of it will be incorporated into the hemoglobin of circulating erythrocytes within seven to ten days. The exact mechanism of the incorporation of iron into hemoglobin remains to be elucidated.

Iron deficiency in adult males and postmenopausal females eating adequate diets is virtually always the result of abnormal blood loss. In the United States, at least, iron deficiency is rarely a purely nutritional disease. When intestinal malabsorption exists for years, as in steatorrhea, iron deficiency may occur on a nutritional basis. Iron deficiency is most commonly seen in females in the reproductive years where the losses of blood from menstruation and the demands for iron associated with childbearing increase the body's demands beyond the ability of a borderline-adequate diet to supply iron. In other societies, iron deficiency on a nutritional basis may persist from childhood into the adult years.

In certain pathological conditions the body's iron stores are vastly increased. Abnormal iron deposits may be seen in many parts of the body. Such a condtiion may be the result of long-continued intake of excessive quantities of iron systemically, as in transfusion hemosiderosis, or in the diet, as in the hemosiderosis of the African Bantu. In the disease hemochromatosis, increased iron deposits are associated with cirrhosis of the liver, fibrosis of the pancreas, and certain endocrine disturbances. This disease appears to be familial, but impressive arguments have been presented that it is only "secondary to conditions and diseases in which there is altered iron metabolism" (R. A. MacDonald, *Prog. Hematol.* **5,** *324 (1966)*). The fundamental biochemical lesion that allows iron to accumulate in the body far in excess of need, and the pathogenesis of the sclerosis of various organs seen in this condition remain unclear.

The importance of copper in human nutrition is uncertain. Clinically apparent copper deficiency has rarely been reported.

Thus the human dietary requirement for copper is not certain. In a small group of malnourished infants, where copper deficiency was seemingly established, it was estimated that the daily requirement for copper of rapidly growing infants was in the range of 42 to 135 μg. per kilogram of body weight (*Nutrition Reviews* **23**, *164* (*1965*)).

It is known that the average diet in the United States contains from 2 to 5 mg. of copper (G. E. Cartwright and M. M. Wintrobe, *Am. J. Clin. Nutrition* **14**, *224* (*1964*)). Of this, from 0.6 to 1.6 mg. are absorbed by the adult. Studies with radioactively labeled copper administered by mouth have revealed that absorbed copper appears rapidly in the plasma bound loosely to albumin, reaching a peak concentration at approximately two hours. There is then some fall in serum copper levels followed by a secondary peak at approximately 24 hours, with the copper then bound tightly to ceruloplasmin, the specific copper-binding protein of plasma. After time for equilibration, as much as 90 per cent of an orally administered dose of copper may be found in the liver. The normal serum copper level is in the range of 90 to 150 μg. per 100 ml. with approximately 90 per cent bound to ceruloplasmin.

Total body copper has been reported to be of the order of 80 mg. Body copper is contained in proteins present in many tissues. Certain of these proteins have known enzymatic activities. These include cytochrome c oxidase, ascorbate oxidase, tyrosinase, and the like. However, these account for only a small amount of total tissue copper. The bulk of tissue copper is to be found in proteins without known enzymatic activities.

The biological actions of copper in the body are not well known. In pigs, experimentally produced copper deficiency is associated with anemia (M. E. Lahey *et al.,*

Blood **7**, *1053* (*1952*); C. J. Gubler *et al., Ibid.* **7**, *1075* (*1952*)). Copper-containing enzymes are frequently found in biological systems having important roles in charge transfer reactions.

Excessive copper appears to be toxic. In experimental animals copper injected directly into the subarachnoid space results in specific types of convulsions. In human beings, certain enzyme systems have been shown to be susceptible to interference by free copper, notably membrane adenosinetriphosphatase and the lipoic acid-pyruvate oxidase system.

A well-known pathological condition in man manifested by excessive body stores of copper is hepatolenticular degeneration, or Wilson's disease. This disease is characterized by a form of neurological degeneration, cirrhosis of the liver, and the presence of corneal pigment rings. Total body stores of copper in Wilson's disease are much increased. Plasma copper levels are reduced, however, and have been shown to be due to reduced levels of ceruloplasmin-bound copper. Much of the copper circulating in the plasma is bound loosely to non-specific proteins, and is therefore much more labile and free to diffuse into the tissues. Elevated urinary levels of copper are seen in Wilson's disease.

It is felt that the primary defect in Wilson's disease may be the failure of the liver to remove albumin-bound copper from the plasma and incorporate the copper into ceruloplasmin. This defect is felt to be due to the genetically determined absence of a liver enzyme system. At the present time, Wilson's disease is treated with chelating agents in an attempt to bind free copper and encourage its excretion from the body. It has been suggested that control of dietary copper may also be of value (*Nutrition Reviews* **23**, *301* (*1965*)).

CHAPTER XXX

PRESENT KNOWLEDGE OF FLUORIDE

JAMES H. SHAW, PH.D.

Rapid progress has been made in knowledge about the effects of human consumption of fluoride on many aspects of health and in application of this knowledge for the benefit of mankind. Various aspects have occupied center stage at different times: 1) recognition in 1931 that excessive ingestion of fluoride during tooth development caused mottled enamel, 2) demonstration from limited field surveys in the United States in the late 1930's that optimal ingestion of fluoride occurring endemically in the water supply during tooth development and maturation resulted in striking reductions in the prevalence of dental caries among children, 3) later demonstration on a wider scale in the United States and many other countries, under a variety of racial, economic, and dietary conditions, that optimal ingestion of fluoride caused major reductions in dental caries prevalence in children which also extended on into adult life, 4) conclusive evidence from laboratory studies, epidemiological surveys, and mortality statistics that ingestion of fluoride at levels optimal for low prevalence of dental caries was not harmful in any way for the human body and did not cause aesthetically undesirable mottled enamel, 5) testing of fluoride additions to communal water supplies (fluoridation) to determine whether the same benefits could be obtained by fortification of low fluoride water supplies, 6) increasing adoption of fluoridation in the United States and in many other countries as an inexpensive, safe, and highly effective public health procedure for reduction of one of the most prevalent and costly chronic diseases.

At the present time about 60,000,000 people in the United States receive water supplies with controlled fluoridation. The most recent, but already outdated, worldwide survey by the Federation Dentaire Internationale in 1963 indicated that controlled fluoridation was in operation or planned at that time in 41 countries.

The benefits of fluoridation of public water supplies have been resoundingly demonstrated in the United States, Canada, the United Kingdom, and Japan. The three benchmark fluoridation projects begun in Brantford, Ontario, Newburgh, N. Y., and Grand Rapids, Mich. in the summer of 1945 have now been in operation for 21 years. Recent data are available for all with comparable results. Only the results of the last Brantford study in 1963 will be summarized here (H. K. Brown and M. Poplove, *J. Canad. Dent. Assn.* **31,** *505* (*1965*)).

Data for the 16 to 17 year olds were of special interest because these individuals had had fluorides at optimal levels throughout their entire lives. The average number of decayed, missing, and filled (DMF) teeth in this population was 4.74 ± 0.18. In Stratford, the city with naturally fluoridated water which served as one control throughout the study, the same age group had 4.19 ± 0.21 DMF teeth. In Sarnia, the control city with the low fluoride water supply, this value was 10.44 ± 0.22. The difference between the values for Sarnia and Brantford was highly significant, while the difference between the values for Brantford and Stratford was not significant. For the same age group, the percentages of individuals who were caries free were 0.41, 11.80, and 21.78 for Sarnia, Brantford, and Stratford, respectively. Very comparable data are available for numerous other communities.

Two other indices of the effectiveness of

water fluoridation, numbers of DMF teeth and percentage of caries free children, have been compiled by D. B. Ast, N. C. Cons, J. P. Carlos, and A. Maiwald (*Am. J. Pub. Health* **55**, *811* (*1965*)) in terms of the chair time and the cost to provide regular periodic dental care for children in the fluoridated area of Newburgh, N. Y., and the non-fluoridated area of Kingston, N. Y. The mean chair time in minutes per child to provide the initial comprehensive dental care upon entrance into school was 76.9 in Newburgh and 117.3 in Kingston. The costs were $14.16 and $32.38, respectively. The mean chair time for incremental yearly dental care after the original rehabilitation was 25.6 minutes per child for Newburgh versus 35.9 minutes per child for Kingston. The mean costs per year were $5.90 and $11.00, respectively. These values reflect very clearly the benefit to be derived from water fluoridation in terms that every dentist or parent, public health worker, or city alderman should be able to understand more readily than figures on dental caries prevalence.

Part-time consumption of water fluoridated at optimal levels during school hours by children who drink low fluoride water at home has been repeatedly shown to cause significant reductions in dental caries prevalence (J. A. Yacovone and V. F. Lisanti, *Arch. Oral Biol.* **1**, *265* (*1960*); *North-West Dent.* **40**, *244* (*1961*); W. A. Jordan, *Ibid.* **41**, *186, 243* (*1962*); W. E. Creighton, J. Savage, and D. M. Witter, *Pub. Health Rep.* **79**, *778* (*1964*). While these reductions were not as great as those with fluoridated water available both at home and at school, the benefits were worthwhile. Many opportunities were available to make these observations in consolidated schools where the town children had a fluoridated water supply while the children from rural areas with private wells had low fluoride water supplies.

Studies have been undertaken to take advantage of fluoride benefits in schools for children from low fluoride areas by providing higher levels of fluoride. H. S. Horowitz, S. B. Heifetz, and F. E. Law (*J. Am. Dent. Assn.* **71**, *1124* (*1965*)) described studies conducted under conditions designed to augment the benefits of part-time consumption in Pike County, Ky., and in Elk Lake, Pa., where the water supplies are not generally fluoridated.

In Pike County the mean maximum daily temperature is 70.3° F. On the basis of this temperature, the optimal fluoride level for a water system used exclusively at home and at school would be 0.9 p.p.m. To take advantage of the part-time situation of the availability of fluoridated water only on school days during school hours, the water supply was fluoridated at a level of 3.0 p.p.m. In Elk Lake, the mean maximum daily temperature was 55.9° F. and the optimal level of fluoride was calculated to be 1.1 p.p.m. for full-time use. Here the water supply was fluoridated at 5.0 p.p.m.

Caries prevalence among children of various ages was evaluated for four years in Elk Lake and five years in Pike County. Good reductions were observed, averaging 24.5 per cent in Elk Lake and 28.0 per cent in Pike County, for all children between six to 17 years of age. The reductions for six year old children only were 59.3 per cent and 51.5 per cent, respectively.

Horowitz, Law, and T. Pritzker (*Pub. Health Rep.* **80**, *381* (*1965*)) made a similar study at a school at St. Thomas in the Virgin Islands, where the mean maximum daily temperature is 84.7° F. and the calculated value for fluoride to produce optimal benefits with full-time use is 0.7 p.p.m. When the water was fluoridated at 2.3 p.p.m. for six years, the 279 children in grades two through seven had 2.47 DMF tooth surfaces, in contrast to a value of 3.21 for the 601 control children. This decrease was significant at a p value <0.001. This procedure may prove to be one way to answer the major problem of the millions of individuals living in homes with private wells and therefore otherwise out of the scope of a communally fluoridated water supply.

The question was often asked in the early years of fluoridation whether other benefits than reduced prevalence of dental caries might result. Information is slowly becoming available in this regard. In three studies in Evanston, Ill., Newburgh, N. Y., and High Point, N. Carolina, separate teams of investigators reported less malocclusion after ten or more years of fluoridation than was true in the same community before fluoridation or in neighboring control communities (I. N. Hill, J. R. Blayney, and W. Wolf, *J. Dent. Res.* **38**, *782* (*1959*); D. B. Ast, N. Allaway, and H. L. Draker, *Am. J. Orth.* **48**, *106* (*1962*); D. M. Erickson and F. W. Graziano, *J. Am. Dent. Assn.* **73**, *124* (*1966*)).

Different methods were used in each of these studies, so they are not strictly comparable. One method of expression used for the Newburgh study was particularly understandable. In Newburgh 9.4 per cent of the children were considered to be physically handicapped by their malocclusion problems, while 22.5 per cent of the children in the non-fluoride community of Kingston were so handicapped. The authors speculated on whether the greater loss of first permanent molars in the control communities contributed to the higher prevalence of malocclusion.

Very similar results were reported in a Japanese study where fluoridation was maintained for 11 years at 0.6 p.p.m. (G. Minoguchi, *Bull. Stomat.* **4**, *45* (*1964*)). The lower level of fluoride in this program was occasioned by the higher level of fluoride in the food of the Japanese than is typical in the United States. The dental benefits with respect to reduced DMF tooth values were good, but slightly lower than for studies in the United States and Canada.

Benefits with regard to the periodontium

have been reported also. H. R. Englander and C. L. White (*Abstracts of the Forty-first General Meeting, International Association for Dental Research,* #262 (*1963*)) compared the periodontal and oral hygiene status of 1,200 lifetime residents of Aurora (1.2 p.p.m. natural fluoride) and 870 similar residents of Rockford (0.1 p.p.m. natural fluoride) in the 13 to 17 year age group. Oral debris, calculus scores, and frequency of tooth brushing were comparable for the two groups. However, the periodontal index was slightly lower for Aurora than for Rockford; a greater proportion of individuals in Aurora was without signs of disease.

The age group from 18 to 65 years was also studied (Englander, R. G. Kesel, and O. P. Gupta (*Abstracts of the Fortieth General Meeting, International Association for Dental Research* #122 (*1962*)). In Aurora 906 white native residents and 950 in Rockford were compared. Periodontal disease was uniformly more severe in the low fluoride city than in the community with an optimal fluoride level in the water. The mean periodontal index was 0.69 in Aurora versus 1.10 in Rockford. This difference was highly significant. Indeed, the difference was more than eight times the standard error of difference in mean scores. Expressed another way, 41 per cent of this group in Rockford had gross periodontal pockets in comparison with 24 per cent in Aurora.

A. L. Russell (*Am. J. Pub. Health* **47**, *688* (*1957*)) compared the prevalence of periodontal disease in Newburgh and Kingston, New York, Colorado Springs and Boulder, Colorado, and Bartlett and Cameron, Texas. In each of the three comparisons, the individuals in the fluoride community had a little less periodontal disease than those in the low fluoride community. He remarked particularly that no evidence whatever was found of the increased periodontal disease in fluoride communities which had been predicted by the opponents of fluoridation.

Repeated demonstrations of the safety of fluoride ingestion at recommended levels have been made over the years. Possibly the weightiest of these was the comparison between citizens of Bartlett, where the water supply contained 8.0 p.p.m. fluoride, and individuals in Cameron, where the water supply contained 0.4 p.p.m. fluoride (*see Nutrition Reviews* **16,** *117* (*1958*)). Two epidemiologic surveys were made in 1943 and 1953. No significant differences between the findings in the two towns were observed except for a slightly higher rate of cardiovascular abnormalities in Cameron and the expected high prevalence and severity of dental fluorosis in Bartlett.

A similar survey has been made in Russia where the fluoride community, Shchuchinsk, had a water supply containing 4 p.p.m. fluoride (V. A. Knizhnikov, *Gigiena i Sanitariya* **23**(*8*), *18* (*1958*)). From the fluoride community, 169 individuals were studied and compared with 53 from the control community, Kokchetav, where several water supplies with fluoride levels varying from 0 to 0.9 p.p.m. were in use. The investigators particularly commented that no differences in such health disorders as spinal rigidity, vegetative dystonia, muscular weakness, anemia, decreased coagubility of blood, and recurrent urticaria were observed between the two communities. He also stated that mortality and morbidity statistics were somewhat more favorable for Shchuchinsk than for Kokchetav. As would be expected, mottled enamel was prevalent among the citizens of Shchuchinsk where 33 per cent had class II and III mottling, but none had the most severe class IV.

Findings were reported on 904 necropsies performed between 1947 and 1953 in Colorado Springs where the water supply contains 2.5 p.p.m. fluoride (*see Nutrition Reviews* **17,** *133* (*1959*)). Of this group, 334 subjects had lived in Colorado Springs for more than 20 years. Evaluation of the pathologic findings revealed no evidence that prolonged exposure to water containing fluoride at this level had been harmful to any organ system.

Many other investigations have been conducted to determine the relationship of fluorides as endemically present or as added in the waterworks to human health. Invariably exhaustive and well documented studies have indicated that ingestion of fluoride from water supplies with recommended levels has been safe over prolonged periods under many climatic and other environmental conditions.

Much effort has been made to evaluate the extent of enamel mottling in communities with optimal fluoride levels in their water supplies. The frequency of mottling and the questionable or very mild (nonesthetically disfiguring) levels have been routinely reported to be around 8 to 10 per cent for children who grew up in the area. Disfiguring mottling has not been observed where recommended levels of fluoridation have prevailed. However, in the political area attendant upon referenda and public hearings, opponents of fluoridation often have distorted the facts about the prevalence and severity of mottling in communities with optimal levels of fluoride in the water supplies.

Additional information is becoming available to establish even more firmly the safety of fluoridation at recommended levels. J. R. Forrest and P. M. C. James (*Brit. Dent. J.* **119,** *319* (*1965*)) had the opportunity to conduct a study of all kinds of enamel opacities on a group of eight year old children who had grown up either in a community with water fluoridation for eight years or in a community with no appreciable fluoride in the water supply. The children were available at one site so that the examiners could perform a detailed inspection of their teeth without knowledge of the community of origin.

When the data were later sorted and compiled, enamel opacities of all kinds were found in 36 per cent of the children from the area with fluoridated water. Of these, 24 per cent had opacities of the idiopathic variety occurring in sites where mottled enamel does not develop or of such a nature that fluoride was not considered to be the cause. The remaining 12 per cent had opacities which could be considered questionable or very mild mottled enamel. Among the children from the low fluoride area, 47 per cent had idiopathic opacities of comparable nature to the 24 per cent from the community with fluoridated water. Many of these opacities were more unsightly than found in children from the fluoride area.

These findings emphasize again the fact that opacities of different types and etiology occur in the enamel. These data emphasize the need for a differential diagnosis among the types of opacities. Benefits of the fluoridation program in this comparison indicated that 38.5 per cent of children from the fluoride area were caries free in comparison with 23.8 per cent for the low fluoride area, and that all four first permanent molars were carious in 12.1 and 27.7 per cent of the children, respectively.

Similar data on mottling were sought among 2,332 children from Meosho, Missouri (<0.1 p.p.m. F), Grand Rapids, Michigan (1.0 p.p.m. F by fluoridation), Grand Prairie, Texas (1.6 to 2.8 p.p.m. F naturally), Bartlett, Texas (8.0 p.p.m. before institution of defluoridation procedures to reduce fluorides to optimal level in 1952) (V. I. Diefenbach, G. A. Nevitt, and J. M. Frankel, *J. Am. Dent. Assn.* **771,** *1129* (*1965*)). They showed that mottled enamel posed no esthetic problem at optimal fluoride levels and indeed that teeth of enhanced appearance occurred more frequently in communities with optimal fluoride, or even with water supplies containing amounts of fluoride beyond those considered optimal, than in low fluoride areas. In the study by Minoguchi (*loc. cit.*) no increase in occurrence of hypoplastic teeth was ob-

served in the fluoridated area. He also commented on the problem of opacities of the enamel in the low fluoride community and had difficulty in differentiating between the types of opacity observed in the two communities.

Progress is steadily being made in the understanding of the relationship of fluoride to bone metabolism (*see Nutrition Reviews* **19,** *198* (*1961*)). During a clinical survey of the health of citizens in Bartlett (8.0 p.p.m. fluoride) and Cameron (0.4 p.p.m. fluoride), roentgenologic evaluations were included. No difference between the communities was noted with respect to the incidence of bone fractures, arthritis, hypertrophic bone changes or exostoses, nor was there any evidence of interference with fracture healing. No cases of "poker back" were observed in either community.

In 15 per cent of the individuals in Bartlett, an increased bone density was observed, either with or without coarsened trabeculation, and an increased thickening of cortical bone and periosteum with questionable narrowing of bone spaces. These changes were slight, often difficult to recognize, and in some cases equivocal in degree. Fewer cases of osteoporosis were observed in Bartlett than in Cameron, which prompted the authors to suggest that fluoride ingestion "may, on occasion, have a beneficial effect on adult bones, as in counteracting the osteoporotic changes of the aged."

Findings were reported of a radiological investigation of 546 persons 30 to 70 years of age who were long term residents of Framingham, Mass. where the water contained only a trace of fluoride. A very high frequency of osteoporosis was observed even in younger age groups, and especially in males. This high prevalence in comparison with the Bartlett-Cameron area suggested the possibility that low fluoride areas might provide inadequate fluoride for maintenance of an adequately mineralized skeleton in middle and advanced age.

Twenty-three cases of osteosclerosis were observed among 170,000 radiologic examinations of patients primarily from Texas and Oklahoma. These patients had nothing in common other than osteosclerosis as radiologically demonstrated. The authors were unable to establish any relationship between the radiologic evidence and the patients' current disease process and symptoms. All 23 patients had had lifetime consumption of water supplies with 4 to 8 p.p.m. fluoride. No osteosclerosis was observed among any of the population groups with less than 4 p.p.m. fluoride.

The prevalence of osteoporosis, reduced bone density, and collapsed vertebrae, and calcification of the abdominal aorta was studied in five communities in North Dakota (see *Nutrition Reviews* **25**, *100* (*1967*)). Brief questionnaires were completed by the subjects and the physician. An x-ray of the lateral lumbar spine was taken of each subject. The high fluoride towns of Mott and Hettinger were in the southwestern part of the state where the drinking water ranged from 5.5 to 5.8 p.p.m. and 4.0 to 4.8 p.p.m., respectively. The low fluoride towns of Grafton, Carrington, and New Rockford were in the northeastern part of the state and had water supplies with fluoride levels ranging from 0.15 to 0.30 p.p.m.

A total of 1,015 individuals of 45 years of age was examined, 300 in the high fluoride towns and 715 in the low fluoride communities. The prevalence of reduced bone density was higher in the low fluoride than in the high fluoride area for all three age groups, 45 to 54, 55 to 64, and 65 and over, and for both sexes. The differences between communities were statistically highly significant (p < 0.01) in the females 55 to 64 and 65 and over age groups and statistically significant (p < 0.05) for males in the 55 to 64 age group.

The corollary was also true: more subjects had normal to increased bone density in the high than in the low fluoride communities. Among the female subjects, a greater prevalence of collapsed vertebrae was observed for the low fluoride than for the high fluoride areas. The same trend was not observed for males in all communities, where an unexpectedly high prevalence of collapsed vertebrae was observed, possibly because the majority were farmers. No difference in the occurrence of osteophytes (bony outgrowths) was observed between the two types of communities.

The history of bone disease, previous hormonal therapy, endocrine abnormalities, age at menopause, and gonadal failure did not differ between the two groups. An unexpected finding was the higher prevalence of aortic calcification among the individuals from the low fluoride communities. The difference was statistically significant for all three age groups among the males. The limited dietary information on the level of dietary calcium as indicated by questions about milk and cheese consumption indicated that calcium intake had not been of etiological significance in the differences of bone density and in the number of collapsed vertebrae.

This survey provides the strongest evidence yet that older individuals in low fluoride communities are at a distinct disadvantage with respect to osteoporosis as indicated by both decreased bone density and collapsed vertebrae. In addition, they may also have a greater frequency of calcification of the abdominal aorta. The high fluoride areas in the survey had fluoride levels well beyond the recommended ones for optimal reductions in tooth decay and minimal occurrence of non-esthetically disfiguring mottled enamel. A comparable survey is needed in areas where water supplies have contained the optimal levels of fluoride for prolonged periods to determine the degree to which the benefits for reduced prevalence of osteoporosis and aortic calcification have been attained.

In recent years, several investigators have been using fairly high levels of fluoride as an experimental procedure for the treatment of metabolic bone disease (M. J. Purves, *Lancet* **2**, *118* (*1962*); D. S. Bernstein *et al.*, *J. Clin. Invest.* **42**, *916* (*1963*); C. Rich, J. Ensinck, and P. Ivanovich, *J. Clin. Invest.* **43**, *545* (*1964*); P. Cohen and F. H. Gardner, *New Engl. J. Med.* **271**, *1129* (*1964*); G. A. Rose, *Proc. Roy. Soc. Med.* **58**, *436*, (*1965*)). Balance studies in the first four of these investigations indicated that the majority of patients with postmenopausal (senile) osteoporosis and Paget's disease went from negative to positive calcium balance during fluoride therapy. In some cases increased bone density was observed in radiologic examination. However, some patients did not respond and in the study by Rose no benefits were observed.

P. Grøn, H. G. McCann, and Bernstein (*J. Bone Joint Surg.* **48-A** *892* (*1966*)) reported the results from examination of 24 iliac crest biopsy specimens from 21 patients. When the biopsy material was compared after treatment with samples before treatment or with samples from untreated individuals, the fluoride content was observed to have increased from 0.087 to 0.35 per cent, the degree of crystallinity of the mineral component was more desirable (Beta = 0.77 as compared with 0.94), and the citrate content was reduced to 1.89 from 2.59 per cent.

Numerous studies have been conducted in recent years to attempt to explain the mechanism of action of fluorides. One of the most interesting of these has come from the demonstration that the hydroxyapatite crystals in bone are larger and more perfectly formed when the fluoride content is higher (*see Nutrition Reviews* **23**, *237* (*1965*)). These studies indicated that with increased fluoride intake during bone mineralization not only the fluoride content increased but the bone mineral crystals were found to have an increased "crystallinity" due to the alterations in crystal size and perfection, which would also result in a reduction in surface area and solubility.

An interesting gradient of fluoride concentration has been reported in the enamel (F. Brudevold, D. E. Gardner, and F. A. Smith, *J. Dent. Res.* **35**, *420* (*1956*); S. Isaac, Brudevold, Smith, and Gardner, *J. Dent. Res.* **37**, *318* (*1958*)). Invariably in high and low fluoride areas and in erupted and unerupted teeth the fluoride concentration in the superficial surface enamel was about ten times higher than in the deeper layers. During the first decade or two after eruption, the fluoride concentration of the surface layer increased significantly. Fluoride has been shown to significantly increase the precipitation of hydroxyapatite crystals from supersaturated solutions of calcium and phosphate in the pH range from 6.2 to 7.4 (Brudevold, B. H. Amdur, and A. Messer, *Arch. Oral Biol.* **6**, *304* (*1961*)).

Numerous studies have been reported in the past decade on the evaluation of fluoride provided in other vehicles such as pills and lozenges, milk, and table salt. B. G. Bibby, E. Wilkins, and E. Witol (*Oral Surg., Oral Med., Oral Path.* **8**, *213* (*1955*)) observed a 30 per cent inhibition of caries after only one year when 1 mg. fluoride per day was administered in lozenges which were dissolved in the mouth before swallowing; no effect was obtained when the same amount of fluoride was given in pills. G. Wrzodek (*Zahnarztl. Mitt.* **7**, *1* (*1959*)) provided fluoride tablets for 13,585 school children in Germany for a period of four years and compared their dental caries incidence with 4,975 children who took no tablets. A 20 per cent reduction in dental caries was observed among first, second, and third grade children.

F. A. Arnold, Jr., F. J. McClure, and C. L. White (*Dent. Prog.* **1**, *8* (*1960*)) gave a fluoride solution and later fluoride tablets to parents who were professional employees of the Public Health Service for their young children. The mean incidence of dental caries of 121 children who took the supplement for an average of two-thirds of their lives was comparable to the incidence for children of similar age who drank fluoridated water. One of the most striking findings was that even among a professional health-oriented group such as this, only about one-half of the parents continued to give their children the fluoride supplement for the necessary number of years.

L. L. Rusoff *et al.* (*Am. J. Clin. Nutrition* **11,** *94* (*1962*)) provided school children with a half-pint of milk containing 1 mg. fluoride in the form of sodium fluoride with their school lunch over a three and one-half year period. At the end of this period, the fluoride group contained 65 children, nine to 12 years of age. Approximately a 70 per cent reduction in caries was observed for the teeth erupting after initiation of fluoridated milk (first and second bicuspids and second molars). A lesser benefit was observed for the first molars, which had erupted just before the beginning of supplementation.

In Switzerland a concentrated effort has been made to use fluoridated table salt, where fluoride is provided at a concentration of 90 p.p.m. (T. M. Marthaler and C. Schenardi, *Helv. Odont. Acta* **6,** *1* (*1962*)). The percentage reduction in carious lesions was 41 for proximal, 32 for buccolabial and 21 for occlusal surfaces after five and one-half years of use. This level of benefit was less than from fluoridated water and the authors proposed that the fluoride level in salt possibly should be increased from 90 to 200 p.p.m.

The data on provision of fluoride through other routes than fluoridation of communal water supplies indicate that worthwhile benefits can be obtained when proper adjustment of fluoride intake is made. However, the success or failure of alternate procedures often turns upon the parent's faithfulness in providing the fluoride source over the necessarily prolonged period.

Much progress has been made during the past decade on the scientific knowledge about fluoride ingestion and human health and in adoption of fluoride supplementation in world-wide scope. With increasing evidence of benefits to man beyond the reduction in tooth decay, we should see a more rapid rate of initiation of fluoridation programs, greater evidence to provide the benefits to individuals beyond the scope of municipal water supplies, and probably the development of higher fluoride levels for adult use than are optimal for children.

Chapter XXXI

PRESENT KNOWLEDGE OF SELENIUM

Orville A. Levander, Ph.D.

Selenium is an unusual mineral, in that natural foods can contain either so much of the element that a toxicosis results or so little that a deficiency occurs. The presence of toxic amounts of selenium in foodstuffs was discovered in the 1930's by workers in the United States who were studying a condition in livestock known as "alkali disease" (I. Rosenfeld and O. A. Beath, *Selenium. Academic Press, New York, 1964*). This malady was shown to be a chronic form of selenium poisoning caused by ingestion of grains and forages containing moderately high levels of selenium (5 to 40 p.p.m.). An acute selenosis, "blind staggers," was observed in animals consuming certain species of plants which are able to accumulate several thousand p.p.m. of selenium. In both of these cases the ultimate source of the selenium was the soil upon which the plants grew and, subsequently, significant quantities of selenium have been found in the soil of several Great Plains and Rocky Mountain regions.

The public health problem of selenium toxicity in agricultural products has been minimized in North America by careful delineation of potentially dangerous seleniferous areas. Unfortunately, such complete data on the geochemical distribution of selenium does not exist in other sectors of the world where there appears to be a possibility of selenium poisoning. In Venezuela, for example, some plant samples of different rural regions contained 10 p.p.m. of selenium (W. G. Jaffé, J. F. Chávez, and M. C. Mondragón, *Arch. Latinamericos Nutricion* **17**, *59* (*1967*)).

Since a concentration of 5 p.p.m. in common foods is considered hazardous, the need

for thorough surveys to assess the magnitude of the problem is clear.

After the initial finding of K. Schwarz and C. M. Foltz (*J. Biol. Chem.* **233**, *245* (*1958*)) that trace quantities of selenium protect against liver necrosis in rats fed *Torula* yeast diets lacking vitamin E, many reports appeared regarding favorable biological effects of minute amounts of selenium. Among the many disorders which have been successfully treated with selenium are infertility, unthriftiness, and white muscle disease in sheep, white muscle disease in calves, *hepatosis diaetetica* in pigs, and exudative diathesis and muscular dystrophy in poultry.

Although the need for selenium seems to be adequately documented for laboratory and farm animals, there is no known corresponding deficiency disease in man. Yet there are some preliminary studies which suggest that selenium deficiency might be a complicating factor in certain types of kwashiorkor. Two Jamaican children suffering from protein malnutrition who did not gain weight after overcoming the initial acute phase responded immediately after receiving daily supplements of 25 μg. selenium as gamma, gamma'-di-seleno-di-valeric acid (Schwarz, *Fed. Proc.* **20**, *666* (*1961*)). A. S. Majaj and L. L. Hopkins, Jr. described malnourished Jordanian infants who showed a striking reticulocyte response after administration of 30 to 50 μg. selenium per day as sodium selenite (*Lancet* **2**, *592* (*1966*)). Majaj and Hopkins also cite work of Viteri, Burke, and W. N. Pearson, who found that selenium levels in the blood of Guatemalan children afflicted with kwashiorkor were about half those of normal children (*First International Symposium on Selenium in Biomedicine. AVI Publishing Co., Westport, Connecticut, 1967*). The promising evidence from these early trials indicates the need for further research regarding the possible role of selenium in human nutrition.

Any attempt to set a selenium requirement must take into account several variables, including the form of dietary selenium itself. Schwarz has repeatedly emphasized that 0.007 p.p.m. of selenium as the naturally occurring organic form ("Factor 3") is the 50 per cent effective dose against liver necrosis in rats, whereas inorganic selenite or selenate is effective only at 0.02 to 0.03 p.p.m. (*Nutrition Reviews* **18**, *193* (*1960*)). M. C. Nesheim and M. L. Scott found that 0.05 to 0.10 p.p.m. of selenium as sodium selenite was needed in a *Torula* yeast diet to prevent exudative diathesis in chicks and turkeys (*Fed. Proc.* **20**, *674* (*1961*)), while J. E. Oldfield, J. R. Schubert, and O. H. Muth were able to eliminate white muscle disease in lambs by feeding their dams prenatally an alfalfa-hay-oats diet containing 0.06 p.p.m. of selenium (*J. Agr. Food Chem.* **11**, *388* (*1963*)).

In regard to human nutrition, it should be pointed out that many organic selenium compounds are quite unstable and are easily lost by heating, so that over-cooking of foods might drive off volatile selenium and thus render diets inadequate in this element. The loss of selenium from heated grains is well known, but few data exist concerning the effect of various processing methods on the selenium content of foods. It is possible that under certain conditions factors known to modify the metabolism of selenium could influence the need of an organism for the element. Linseed oil meal counteracts chronic selenium toxicity (A. W. Halverson, C. M. Hendrick, and O. E. Olson, *J. Nutrition* **56**, *51* (*1955*)) and might affect the selenium balance in an animal, and recently arsenic has been shown to increase biliary excretion of selenium under a wide variety of conditions (O. A. Levander and C. A. Baumann, *Toxicol. Appl. Pharmacol.* **9**, *106* (*1966*)).

Addition of selenium to foodstuffs for animals or humans should be done with caution until the controversial status of the element as a possible carcinogen is completely clarified. The first report of selenium as a potential cancer inducing agent was that of A. A. Nelson, O. G. Fitzhugh, and H. O. Calvery, who fed seleniferous wheat and $(KNH_4S)_5Se$ in life-term rat studies, and saw adenomas or low grade carcinomas in 11 of 53 rats surviving more than 18 months (*Cancer Res.* **3**, *230* (*1943*)). Similar results were obtained by L. A. Cherkes, S. G. Aptekar, and M. N. Volgarev, who fed sodium selenate and found tumors in ten out of 23 rats living 18 months (*Biull. Eksp. Biol. Med.* **3**, *78* (*1962*)).

However, this work has been criticized by D. V. Frost (*World's Poultry Sci. J.* **21**, *139* (*1965*)), and a rather complete study involving almost 1,500 rats fed several levels of sodium selenite or selenate over a period of three and one-half years led to the conclusion that "no neoplasms found could be attributable to selenium" (J. R. Harr *et al.*, *First International Symposium on Selenium in Biomedicine*). Although this would seem to indicate the non-carcinogenicity of dietary selenite and selenate in rats, the possibility of tumor-producing organic forms of selenium or of selenium producing tumors in other species cannot be excluded.

The function of selenium in cellular metabolism remains a mystery. The many nutritional interrelationships between selenium and vitamin E, and the demonstrated activity of several selenium compounds as effective antioxidants and radioprotective agents *in vitro*, constitute the basis for the theory that the sole metabolic action of selenium is that of a nonspecific antioxidant (A. L. Tappel, *Fed. Proc.* **24**, *73* (*1965*)). However, there are a number of typical vitamin E deficiencies which do not respond to treatment with selenium, such as resorption sterility in rats, muscular dystrophy in rabbits, and encephalomalacia in chicks, and this has convinced other workers that, while selenium may act as an antioxidant in some cases, there is sufficient evidence to suggest a more subtle role for the element. I. D. Desai, C. C. Calvert, and Scott performed a time sequence study of the interrelationships of peroxidation, lysosomal enzymes, and nutritional muscular dystrophy in the chick, and concluded that increased susceptibility of muscle lipids to peroxidation and increased lysosomal enzyme activity are not the primary abnormalities responsible for the onset of muscular dystrophy (see Nutrition Reviews 23, 90 (1965)).

Schwarz has postulated that vitamin E and selenium have independent effects in alternate pathways of metabolism and that this explains why the absence of both nutrients is necessary to develop certain deficiency states (Fed. Proc. 24, 58 (1965)). He has also presented work which indicates that the ability of selenium, sulfur amino acids, and tocopherol to halt the development of respiratory decline in rat liver slices could be rationalized by considering the effects of these materials on one enzyme system, α-ketoglutarate oxidase. That selenium may have an effect independent of vitamin E is also supported by the data of Nesheim and Scott, who showed a growth stimulating activity of selenium in chicks receiving adequate amounts of vitamin E (Ibid. 20, 674 (1961)). Lastly, there is the intriguing report of J. Pinsent that traces of selenite and molybdate are essential for the production of the enzyme formic dehydrogenase in Escherichia coli (Biochem. J. 57, 10 (1954)). This experiment suggests a role for selenium in protein biosynthesis which might have important consequences in mammalian systems.

CHAPTER XXXII

PRESENT KNOWLEDGE OF ZINC IN NUTRITION

W. G. HOEKSTRA, PH.D.

About 30 years ago, zinc was recognized as a dietary essential for laboratory animals and as a component of the enzyme, carbonic anhydrase. Because of the abundance of zinc in foods and feedstuffs relative to the apparent requirement of the laboratory rat and mouse, it was surmised that this element was easily procured in the diet, and not a practical nutritional problem.

That this is definitely not the case has been conclusively demonstrated. In fact, in certain species zinc deficiency is not uncommon, primarily because of restricted availability of dietary zinc.

Relatively recent, comprehensive reviews on zinc in nutrition and metabolism have been published (B. L. Vallee, *Physiol. Reviews* **39**, *443* (*1959*); *Mineral Metabolism*, C. L. Comar and F. Bronner, Editors, Vol. II, Part B, p. *443*. Academic Press, New York, 1962; E. J. Underwood, *Trace Elements in Human and Animal Nutrition*, Second Edition, p. *157*. Academic Press, New York, 1962; Zinc Metabolism, A. S. Prasad, Editor. Charles C Thomas, Springfield, Illinois, 1966). Zinc deficiency was first unequivocally demonstrated in rats and mice. The principal gross symptoms are reduced growth, abnormal hair coat, depigmentation of dark haired strains, alopecia, and scaliness, particularly of the tail. More detailed histologic studies (R. H. Follis, Jr., in *Zinc Metabolism*, p. **129**) have revealed, as direct effects of zinc deficiency and not inanition, hyperkeratinization and thickening of the epidermis with loss of hair follicles and extensive parakeratosis of the esophagus. In severe zinc deficiency in young male rats sterility from testicular atrophy (due to zinc deficiency *per se*) and decreased size of accessory sex organs (due to inadequate gonadotrophin output) have been described (M. J. Millar, P. V. Elcoate, M. L. Fischer, and C. A. Mawson, *Canad. J. Biochem. Physiol.* **38**, *1457* (*1960*)).

In early work, special and time-consuming "purifying" of dietary components to remove zinc was necessary to produce the deficiency. Severe zinc deficiency can now be produced with semipurified diets by reasonable care in selecting cages and dietary ingredients to minimize zinc contamination and by using an appropriate, commercially available protein or amino acid source, such as salt free casein hydrolyzate (zinc is removed during hydrolysis, neutralization, and removal of salts), isolated soybean protein (zinc is of low availability) or dried egg white (naturally very low in zinc; excess biotin must be used or the avidin destroyed). Zinc deficiency was reported to develop in newborn mice deprived of colostrum, but apparently these observations have not been extended.

H. C. H. Kernkamp and E. F. Ferrin (*J. Am. Vet. Med. Assn.* **123**, *217* (*1953*)) described a disease of swine characterized by a dermatitis and poor growth, which they called parakeratosis (occurrence of cell nuclei or nuclear remnants in the outermost layers of the epidermis), and postulated that it was of nutritional origin. The first evidence that zinc might be of value in counteracting parakeratosis (J. T. Raper and L. V. Curtin, in *Proceedings of the Third Conference on Processing as Related to Nutritive Value of Cottonseed Meal, p. 17. 1953*) and that calcium or phosphorus aggravated this dermatitis (N. R. Ellis,

141

Ibid, p. 16) appeared in a publication of limited circulation and was not sufficiently conclusive. H. F. Tucker and W. D. Salmon (*see Nutrition Reviews* **13,** *303* (*1955*)) published unequivocal evidence that zinc dramatically cured or prevented parakeratosis in pigs and that a calcium and phosphorus supplement aggravated the condition. These observations were confirmed by many workers, and it was shown that, in swine fed practical diets, calcium, not phosphorus, was the antagonist to zinc; phosphorus supplements without calcium moderated the dermatitis but did not stimulate growth.

Although there has been some question whether parakeratosis is solely a nutritional problem (*see* I. Mansson, *Acta Vet. Scandinav.* **5,** *279, 287, 295, 305* (*1964*)), production of a similar syndrome with semipurified diets low in zinc (W. H. Smith, M. P. Plumlee, and W. M. Beeson, *J. Animal Sci.* **20,** *128* (*1961*)) is rather conclusive evidence that the naturally occurring disease is indeed a zinc deficiency "conditioned" by factors that reduce availability of dietary zinc.

Shortly after, it was found that zinc was responsible, at least in part, for the "unknown growth factor" response in chicks and turkey poults fed isolated soybean protein diets (B. L. O'Dell and J. E. Savage, *Poultry Sci.* **36,** *459* (*1957*)). More severe forms of zinc deficiency were subsequently produced experimentally in chicks, turkey poults, hens (*Nutrition Reviews* **19,** *111, 148, 302* (*1958*); E. W. Kienholz, M. L. Sunde, and W. G. Hoekstra; *J. Nutrition* **75,** *211* (*1961*)), and Japanese quail (M. R. Spivey Fox and B. N. Harrison, *Proc. Soc. Exp. Biol. Med.* **116,** *256* (*1964*)).

The primary symptoms in young birds made deficient after normal hatching are decreased growth, "frizzled" feathers, moderate but usually not severe hyperkeratosis, labored respiration (not always observed), and often a "perosis-like" or "arthritic-like" leg deformity characterized by enlargement of the hock joint, shortening and thickening of the long bones, and unsteady gait. Some histopathological observations have been made on zinc deficient chicks (O'Dell, P. M. Newberne, and Savage, *J. Nutrition* **65,** *503* (*1958*); R. J. Young, H. M. Edwards, Jr., and M. B. Gillis, *Poultry Sci.* **37,** *1100* (*1958*)). Not all low zinc diets cause the leg deformity in chicks. With soy protein diets leg deformities due to zinc deficiency are a consistent finding.

However, when diets containing salt free, acid-hydrolyzed casein or spray dried egg white were used in place of soy protein, severe zinc deficiency resulted but leg deformities were absent. Moreover, the leg deformity, but not the growth defect, caused by low zinc, soy protein diets has been prevented by a high level (1 to 2 per cent) of dietary histidine or by feeding a lower level (0.2 per cent) of histamine (F. H. Nielsen, M. L. Sunde, and Hoekstra, *Proc. Soc. Exp. Biol. Med.* **48,** *521* (*1967*)). The relationship of zinc deficiency to histamine is not yet understood, but it may have implications in the zinc deficiency syndrome in other species.

Hens fed zinc deficient soy protein diets for several months do not appear grossly deficient; however, chicks and embryos produced from such hens show pronounced defects. A mild zinc deficiency causes weak chicks, which show labored respiration and refusal to eat, and die within a day or two. More severe deficiency produces low hatchability and embryo malformations, primarily skeletal, of which "rumplessness," smallness of limbs, absence of limbs, spinal deformities, and absence of vertebral development are most common. Absence or smallness of eyes, edematous swelling of the muscles of the neck, and beak deformities are sometimes observed, but visceral development is almost always normal.

Experimental zinc deficiency in lambs and calves is characterized primarily by poor growth, anorexia, depraved appetite, dermatitis (hyperkeratosis and parakeratosis with open lesions and swelling above the hoofs) alopecia and swelling with stiffness of joints. Syndromes in cattle ascribed to zinc deficiency have been reported. The incidence in ruminants is presently unknown, but it would not appear to be widespread. Zinc deficiency has also been produced in dogs.

A. S. Prasad and co-workers (*see Zinc Metabolism, p. 250*) have implicated zinc deficiency in human patients in Egypt who show dwarfism, hypogonadism, and hepatosplenomegaly. A similar condition seen in Iran was also believed to result from zinc deficiency. In comparison with control subjects, dwarfs were observed to have low serum zinc concentrations and low urinary zinc excretion; they also cleared injected ^{65}Zn from plasma more rapidly and excreted less in the urine. Effects of zinc supplementation without the other dietary changes accompanying hospitalization were not reported. However, considerable evidence was published that zinc supplementation stimulated growth more than did simple dietary change from a "village diet" to a hospital diet and supplementation with iron.

Two patients who refused treatment and returned to their villages failed to grow. Moreover, zinc promoted development of pubic hair and growth of the external genitalia and the size of the liver and spleen usually decreased, effects which were not seen during the same time period from iron supplementation and change to the hospital diet.

Dwarfs from Iran were known to practice geophagia (clay eating) while the Egyptians dwarfs did not. The diet of Egyptian dwarfs was largely bread and beans (from which zinc may be poorly available) and they commonly had hookworm infection. While an impressive amount of evidence has been accumulated, particularly with the Egyptian dwarfs, that such patients are zinc deficient, it has not been clearly shown whether zinc deficiency *per se* was the cause

or whether it is an abnormality associated with other aspects of nutrition, disease, or metabolism. Moreover, it is not known how prevalent this condition is or whether a milder form of zinc deficiency is of common occurrence.

W. H. Strain *et al.* (*J. Lab. Clin. Med.* **68**, *244* (*1966*)) showed low levels of zinc in the hair of the Egyptian dwarfs and a response of hair zinc to dietary zinc supplementation was demonstrated. Six persons from Rochester, N. Y. had levels of hair zinc which these authors considered to be below "normal" in the winter months but not in summer months. To ascertain whether this bears any relationship to dietary zinc status and whether it indicates a need for zinc supplementation requires more study.

Zinc deficiency in animals and apparently in man has been explained largely by other dietary factors which decrease availability of dietary zinc. Of these, calcium and phytate have been most extensively studied. The effect of excess calcium in aggravating zinc deficiency has often been dramatic; it appears to be most prominent in the pig, and has also been demonstrated in chicks, hens, rats, and dogs but apparently is not documented for ruminants.

Phytate has been shown to decrease zinc availability in chicks, pigs, and rats and a calcium:phytate:zinc interaction has been demonstrated (H. J. A. Likuski and R. M. Forbes, *J. Nutrition* **85**, *230* (*1965*); D. Oberleas, M. E. Muhrer, and B. L. O'Dell, *J. Nutrition* **90**, *56* (*1966*)). In these studies calcium was antagonistic to zinc only in the presence of rather large amounts of dietary phytate. The calcium-phytate complex apparently acted to complex zinc in the intestinal tract into an unavailable form.

Studies with rats using ^{65}Zn indicated that, with a practical diet (containing phytate), calcium decreased zinc absorption. A similar effect was observed with a semipurified diet (free of phytate) *only* when the dietary phosphate level was high (about

1 per cent P) (D. A. Heth, W. M. Becker, and Hoekstra, *J. Nutrition* **88**, *331* (*1966*)). A reasonable concept at present is that calcium antagonizes zinc primarily at the site of intestinal absorption, but that such effects are observed only when an anionic material such as phytate or phosphate persists in rather large amounts in the intestine to combine with calcium and form a complex that firmly binds zinc.

Such binding effects on zinc have been shown *in vitro* both with phosphate (P. K. Lewis, Jr., R. H. Grummer, and Hoekstra, *J. Animal Sci.* **16**, *927* (*1957*)) and with phytate (C. A. Byrd and G. Matrone, *Proc. Soc. Exp. Biol. Med.* **119**, *347* (*1965*)). Certain other phosphate complexes have also been shown to reduce zinc availability (P. Vohra and F. H. Kratzer, *J. Nutrition* **89**, *106* (*1966*)). The above considerations may be used to explain the observation that in an experiment with human subjects (H. Spencer, V. Vankinscott, I. Lewin, and J. Samachson, *J. Nutrition* **86**, *169* (*1965*)), and in some animal experiments, calcium antagonism of zinc was not observed. The reported alleviation of mild parakeratosis in pigs by either zinc or high levels of soybean oil may be the result of formation of calcium soaps, thus reducing calcium antagonism of zinc; this possibility apparently has not been studied.

Vitamin D has also been implicated as a factor affecting zinc availability, paradoxically in decreasing and in stimulating zinc absorption. Recent work (W. M. Becker and Hoekstra, *J. Nutrition* **90**, *301* (*1966*)) indicates that vitamin D probably has no direct role in stimulating intestinal absorption of zinc as it does calcium, but that by causing more zinc to become deposited in bone which has suddenly been stimulated to grow and calcify, it may indirectly (by a homeostatic mechanism) increase zinc absorption. Vitamin D, whether absent, present in required amounts, or present in excess, has not significantly aggravated or alleviated the zinc deficiency syndrome in either swine or rats.

Cadmium has been shown a zinc antagonist, probably by replacing zinc at important sites in the body (J. Pařízek, *J. Reprod. Fertil.* **1**, *294* (*1960*); S. A. Gunn, T. C. Gould, and W. A. D. Anderson, *Arch. Path.* **71**, *274* (*1961*); W. C. Supplee, *Science* **139**, *119* (*1963*); *Nutrition Reviews* **19**, *340* (*1961*)). A practical problem of dietary cadmium antagonizing zinc has not been unequivocally demonstrated; however, intakes of low levels of cadmium over long periods of time have been implicated by H. A. Schroeder and co-workers in decreasing life span of rats and mice and of causing various metabolic defects (such as hypertension) in laboratory animals and possibly in man (*see Nutrition Reviews* **20**, *25* (*1962*); **21**, *340* (*1963*)). Whether such defects can be prevented by increasing the supply of zinc has not yet been demonstrated.

Because high levels of dietary zinc cause a relative copper deficiency it might be expected that copper might be a zinc antagonist. One report suggests that this may be the case (P. J. O'Hara, A. P. Newman, and R. Jackson, *Aust. Vet. J.* **36**, *225* (*1960*)), but most indicate that copper either has no effect on zinc deficiency or alleviates it. This puzzling situation has not been explained.

Protein source has a marked effect on zinc requirements, with soy protein and sesame meal causing a much higher zinc requirement than casein or egg white (*Nutrition Reviews* **19**, *111* (*1961*); R. M. Forbes and J. M. Yohe, *J. Nutrition* **70**, *52* (*1960*)). Such effects have been blamed on the phytic acid content of plant seed proteins, but at present this does not seem to be satisfactory as a sole explanation for the effects of such protein sources. Heating by autoclaving improves zinc availability from such proteins. Many, but not all, dietary chelating agents, such as ethylenediamine tetraacetic acid, have been shown to alleviate zinc deficiency produced by feeding soy protein (Vohra and Kratzer, *J. Nutrition* **82**, *249* (*1964*)). The effect has been postulated to be through the chelators having sufficient zinc binding affinity to remove zinc from complexes with materials like phytate, and to render the zinc in an absorbable form. Effects of possible natural chelators (*i.e.*, amino acids, proteins, and the like) have not been widely studied. However, cysteine (but not cystine) has been reported to alleviate all symptoms of zinc deficiency in chicks fed soy protein while histidine alleviated only the leg abnormality.

In swine, the combination of feeding the diet in a freshly moistened form and limiting food intake to a one hour period twice a day (compared with ad libitum feeding) has been effective in alleviating zinc deficiency (P. K. Lewis, Jr., R. H. Grummer, and Hoekstra, *J. Animal Sci.* **16**, *927* (*1957*)). Such an effect does not appear to have been studied in other species, and its mechanism has not been demonstrated. It is cited to stress the point that rather subtle dietary changes can markedly affect zinc requirements.

In view of the many interactions of zinc with other dietary components, it is apparent that statements of zinc requirements cannot be made without defining the specific dietary conditions. Recent estimates of the zinc requirement range from about 12 p.p.m. of the air-dry diet for young rats fed a casein diet to more than 70 p.p.m. zinc for young turkey poults and pigs fed practical diets. Zinc requirements of adults are less than for young growing animals, but detailed requirements have not been formulated. The zinc requirement for man is not known, but from balance studies the requirement has recently been tentatively estimated for preadolescent girls to be about 6 mg. zinc per day (R. W. Engel, R. F. Miller, and N. O. Price, in *Zinc Metab-*

olism, p. 326) which is not in serious disagreement with earlier estimates. It would not appear difficult to achieve such intakes with a wide variety of diets, but in view of the experiences with animals fed different types of diet, more work is needed with human subjects before zinc requirements are adequately assessed.

Zinc is a component of numerous metalloenzymes, including animal sources of carbonic anhydrase, alkaline phosphatases, pancreatic carboxypeptidases A and B, alcohol deydrogenase, lactate dehydrogenase, glutamate dehydrogenase, glyceraldehyde-3-phosphate dehydrogenase, and malate dehydrogenase. Recognition of zinc as an integral part of numerous enzymes has adequately explained why it is a required element; however, the critical sites of metabolic defect in zinc deficient animals are unknown. Generally, there is little or no decrease in the zinc concentration of most organs or tissues of zinc deficient animals compared with animals receiving sufficient, but not excess, zinc. Among exceptions are bone, hair, feathers, blood plasma, egg yolks, and sometimes pancreas, liver and testes. The pool of rapidly turning-over zinc in the body appears to be decreased in zinc deficiency.

Attempts to find decreases in specific zinc metalloenzymes, such as the dehydrogenases, in most soft tissues of zinc deficient animals have usually failed. Blood plasma alkaline phosphatase usually decreases in zinc deficiency, but the metabolic significance of this decrease is unknown. Surprisingly, a rather marked decrease in soft tissue zinc concentration has been reported in vitamin B_6 deficient rats, but the cause and implication of this effect are unsettled and it has not been studied in other species (J. M. Hsu, *Proc. Soc. Exp. Biol. Med.* **119**, *177* (*1965*)).

Fasted zinc deficient rats have been reported to oxidize ^{14}C labeled carbohydrate and fat substrates like fasted control rats, but a greater proportion of a dose of labeled amino acids was oxidized to respiratory CO_2 by zinc deficient rats (R. C. Theuer and Hoekstra, *J. Nutrition* **89,** *448* (*1966*)). This, and studies with simpler organisms or systems has led to the speculation that energy metabolism is not substantially deranged in zinc deficient animals but that some aspect of protein metabolism, nucleic acid metabolism, or cell division is defective. The specific role of zinc in these processes has not been elucidated. This idea, however, is consistent with the marked effect of zinc deficiency on growth. Turk (*Poultry Sci.* **45,** *608* (*1966*)) recently reported no alteration in liver content of DNA, RNA, total nitrogen, or acid soluble nitrogen of zinc deficient chicks.

Among other defects in zinc deficient animals are delayed and irregular glucose and amino acid absorption and decreased pancreatic amylase and proteolytic activity (rat), decreased pancreatic carboxypeptidase A, but not B (rat), increased blood uric acid (rat), although this was not confirmed in a recent study (M. H. Macapinlac, W. N. Pearson, and W. J. Darby, in *Zinc Metabolism, p. 142*); increased blood plasma gammaglobulin with or without decreased albumin (swine, lambs, and calves), decrease in a specific blood lipoprotein with prolonged fasting (quail), decreased serum alkaline phosphatase (swine, calves, and man), decreased intestinal alkaline phosphatase (rat), and decreased bone alkaline phosphatase (poult). Whether such effects result directly from zinc deficiency or indirectly from inanition, poor food intake, or susceptibility to infection has often not been delineated.

Possible relationships of zinc to insulin storage or release have been widely studied, but the data are not conclusive. Observations made on a role of zinc in stimulating the healing of wounds in rats and man (W. J. Pories and Strain, in *Zinc Metabolism,*

p. 378) and on defective wound healing in zinc deficient calves (W. J. Miller, J. D. Morton, W. J. Pitts, and C. M. Clifton, *Proc. Soc. Exp. Biol. Med.* **118,** *427* (*1965*)) deserve further study. The study of zinc in body tissues has been greatly aided by the development of accurate methods of analysis. Atomic absorption spectrophotometry is a recent important development in this field. Diseases consistently associated with alterations in zinc metabolism are: postalcoholic cirrhosis (decreased serum zinc, decreased liver zinc, increased urinary zinc excretion); pernicious anemia (increased zinc content of red blood cells); and chronic myeloid leukemia (decreased zinc content of granulocytes) (Prasad, in *Zinc Metabolism, p. 250*). A recent report indicated a more generalized decrease in zinc content of granulocytes, as evaluated histochemically in the blood stream or bone marrow, in a wide variety of neoplastic diseases, but more data are needed to support this contention (W. P. Lawkowicz, I. I. Kszeminska-Lawkowicz, S. Szmigolski, and I. Litwin, *Fed. Proc.* **25,** *part II, T809* (*1966*)). Zinc content of serum has been reported to decrease in many acute and chronic infections and to correlate with fever, but the validity of this observation has been questioned. Zinc deficiency may also be associated with kwashiorkor (H. H. Sandstead *et al., Am. J. Clin. Nutrition* **17,** *15* (*1965*)).

The literature abounds with reports of altered zinc concentrations or metabolism in many diseases which are often unconfirmed or controversial. With many diseases, and in particular with reference to neoplastic diseases, it is not possible at present to make a general statement on the relationship to zinc metabolism. The fact that many diseases have been reported to alter blood and other tissue zinc concentrations, however, must be considered in nutritional investigations.

Chapter XXXIII

PRESENT KNOWLEDGE OF CALCIUM, PHOSPHORUS, AND MAGNESIUM

D. M. Hegsted, Ph.D.

Calcium and phosphorus together constitute the major part of the mineral content of skeletal tissues. Most of the body's calcium (99 per cent) and phosphorus (70 to 80 per cent) are in the bones and the ratio of one to the other, while not entirely constant, is nearly so. Appreciable losses or gains by the body of one of these elements may be expected to be reflected in similar changes in the other.

This high mineral content is largely responsible for the rigidity and strength of the bones and teeth. Bones constitute a mineral reserve which may be drawn upon in time of need. The more easily mobilized calcium is in the trabeculae; hard tissues of the teeth, dentine and enamel, are more metabolically stable.

Calcium

W. F. Neuman and M. W. Neuman (*The Chemical Dynamics of Bone Mineral. University of Chicago Press, Chicago, 1958*) give the overall composition of bone mineral (primarily hydroxy apatite crystals) as:

$$[Ca_9^{++} (H_3O^+)_2 (PO_4^\equiv)_6 (OH)_2^-]$$

$$[Ca^{++} \cdot Mg_{0.3}^{++} \cdot Na_{0.3}^+ \cdot CO_3^\equiv \cdot cit_{0.3}^\equiv]$$

Since there appears to be no evidence of more than one phase, it is assumed that the exact composition is determined by surface exchange. Recent evidence leads to the conclusion that normal serum is actually supersaturated with respect to bone mineral. Thus the problem has shifted from explaining mechanisms which cause calcification to discovering those systems which prevent and control calcium deposition.

Since the fluid bathing the crystals cannot be supersaturated, the interstitial fluid cannot be the same as serum. The presence of such materials as carbonate, Mg^{++}, Na^+, citrate, pH, and the like, greatly modifies the solubility of bone hydroxy apatite. Regulatory mechanisms such as those involving vitamin D and the parathyroid presumably act by modifying cellular activity which produces materials that modify solubility and thus maintain a gradient between the interstitial fluid and serum.

Bone formation is dependent upon the activity of osteoblasts which synthesize the organic matrix and presumably modify the calcification process. The chemistry and biochemistry of polysaccharides and cartilagenous proteins is now being actively investigated. It suffices to say here that the familiar tendency of many to equate bone disease with abnormalities in calcium metabolism has little to recommend it.

It should be possible, by utilizing the radioactive isotopes which are metabolized in a manner very similar to calcium, to trace the movement of calcium in various tissues. However, interpretation of isotopic studies has been more complicated than at first anticipated (*see* R. P. Heaney, *Clin. Orth.* **31**, *153* (*1963*)). Neuman and Neuman list the following factors which influence the entrance and fate of ions entering the mineral phase of bone:

Physiochemical mechanisms: a) new crystal formation; b) recrystallization; c) surface exchange; d) intracrystalline exchange (diffusion into the crystal interior); and e) crystal growth.

Physiologically modifying influences:

a) matrix formation b) resorption of bone; c) maturity of bone (the age determines rates of diffusion, recrystallization, and the like); and d) regulatory factors, such as excretion rates, parathyroid function, vitamin D, and dilution by dietary materials.

Within a few minutes to perhaps an hour, injected radiocalcium equilibrates with the "rapidly miscible pool," which includes calcium in plasma and extracellular fluid and some of the calcium in cells and bone. Over a day or two it mixes with the "total miscible pool," which contains an additional fraction of bone and cellular calcium, and that in cartilage and calcified soft tissues. Approximately 100 to 200 mg. of calcium are thought to be excreted into the gut, partially diluted by dietary calcium and partly reabsorbed. The radiocalcium is further diminished by urinary excretion and formation of new "non-exchangeable bone." Over longer periods, bone resorption will further dilute the miscible pool.

Ideally, the objective is to be able to measure the size of each component of the pools and the rates of exchange between them. When modifications in calcium metabolism occur, these should characterize the nature of the abnormality. Calcium-47, a gamma emitter, is available, and deposition in bone in different areas may now be estimated by external counting.

Deposition of radiocalcium in bone is not synonymous with bone growth because of the exchange at the crystal surface. It seems clear that the exchangeable fraction is about 5 per cent of the total bone in young animals and much less in adult animals. Calcium deficiency appears to increase the exchangeable fraction. This is probably part of the adaptive process which favors calcium retention when the intake is low.

In the serum, the level of calcium is controlled by the parathyroid and is not easily changed by variations in the calcium intake. The parathyroid hormone controls the serum level by direct action upon bone and indirectly by modifying the renal excretion of phosphate. Recent evidence indicates the presence of additional parathyroid hormones, calcitonin and thyrocalcitonin, which oppose the effects of conventional parathormone (D. H. Copp et al., Endocrinology 70, 638 (1962)).

The normal serum calcium level is about 10 mg. per 100 ml. (5.0 mEq per liter). About 60 per cent of this is usually ionized and most of the remainder is bound to serum proteins. The degree of ionization is largely dependent upon protein concentration and pH. The level of ionized calcium is important in maintaining the functional integrity of many cells, especially normal neuromuscular irritability. A substantial decrease results in tetany while an increase may lead to respiratory or cardiac failure through impaired muscle function. However, change in the level of dietary calcium is rarely the cause of such conditions in man.

In vitro studies of calcium absorption utilizing gut loops have demonstrated that calcium can be absorbed against a concentration gradient by an energy requiring process dependent upon or stimulated by vitamin D administration. The efficiency of the process is dependent upon the calcium content of the diet and parathormone action (L. B. Dowdle, D. Schachter, and H. Schwenker, Am. J. Physiol. 198, 269 (1960)). Calcium may also be absorbed by simple diffusion, and this may also be dependent on vitamin D (H. E. Harrison and H. C. Harrison, Ibid. 199, 265 (1960)). It is possible that the active process might be essentially a reserve mechanism being called into play when calcium supplies are short and suppressed when supplies are abundant.

The effects of phosphates, phytates, and oxalates as inhibitors of calcium absorption have been demonstrated in experimental animals and in certain situations in man. It seems unlikely, however, that these materials are ordinarily important determinants of the calcium requirement of man. The

FAO-WHO Report (*Calcium Requirements. World Health Organization Technical Report Series No. 230, Geneva, 1961*) points out that some high vegetable diets contain sufficient phytate to theoretically precipitate all the dietary calcium, yet habitual consumers of such diets are not known to suffer from lack of calcium. Absorption of the phosphorus present as phytate presumably requires hydrolysis by phytase and there have been numerous attempts to determine whether intestinal phytase is of endogenous or dietary origin. Oxalates might be expected to seriously inhibit calcium absorption in view of the very low solubility of calcium oxalate. There appears, however, to be no evidence that the ordinary levels in human diets are particularly important.

Considerable evidence indicates that certain amino acids, citric acid, and lactose, may enhance calcium absorption in animals. Whether any of these effects is sufficiently striking or prolonged to be of importance in human nutrition is unknown and seems unlikely to be so.

Calcium is poorly utilized in the steatorrheas. Whether the loss of calcium is caused by the high level of free fatty acids and the insolubility of calcium soaps or the more direct result of the disease and its complications appears uncertain.

The effect of the emotions on calcium balance may be most interesting when adequate data are available. O. Malm (*Calcium Requirement and Adaptation in Adult Men. Oslo University Press, Oslo, 1958*) described a subject on an intake of 574 mg. per day, in positive balance, who retained 60 mg. per day. During the following 10 months, with increasing worry and tension, he was consistently in negative balance, reaching at one point −921 mg. per day. With removal of the tension, balance improved markedly.

Increased attention should be paid to excretion of calcium in sweat, traditionally assumed to be an insignificant quantity. There are, however, data to the contrary. C. F. Consolazio et al. (*J. Nutrition* **78**, 78 (*1962*)) have calculated losses as high as 1 g. per day in individuals working at high temperatures where sweating is profuse.

Most of the calcium in the feces is unabsorbed dietary calcium, but some is of endogenous origin. It is generally thought that there is no active excretion into the gut, but rather that calcium in intestinal secretions becomes mixed with dietary calcium and its reabsorption follows that of dietary calcium. Fecal excretions substantially above the total dietary intake have been recorded. Whether such situations reflect failure of absorptive mechanisms or increased fecal excretion remains to be studied.

The level of calcium in the urine appears to be in large part dependent upon endogenous factors characteristic of the individual, other factors being equal. Increases in calcium absorption, for example, will raise the level of excretion, but the baseline of excretion remains different in different individuals. Age and sex are not important variables, if excretion is expresed on a unit weight basis.

In considering calcium requirements, it is worthwhile to point out the often ignored fact that calcium balances are likely to be poor estimates of actual calcium retention. Since the "balance" is the difference between a large intake and a large excretion, the difference between these is inherently inaccurate. The usual errors, failure of the subject to consume all of the diet and failure to collect all of the excreta, lead to false positive balances. The extent to which such errors have influenced current thinking is unknown.

Estimates of the calcium requirements for infants and children have been derived by calculation of the rates of skeletal growth from body weight changes. The infant starts life with approximately 30 g. of body calcium and the adult body may be assumed to have 1,000 to 1,200 g. An assumed intake of 0.5 g. per day which is 30 per cent utilized would yield 1,000 g. of body calcium in 20 years. The Recommended Dietary Allowances are thus substantially above theoretical estimates of need. The WHO-FAO suggested practical allowances, however, approximate this estimate.

Contrary to the situation in children where calcium retention is necessary, the well-nourished adult has no apparent need for more calcium than that required to maintain body stores. Average intake in countries where milk is not a common food and where there are no other unusual sources of calcium is probably of the order of 300 to 400 mg. per day, yet the adults remain in balance. Adults are found on the average to be in balance at the level of intake supplied by their usual diet. Hence the author has concluded that ordinarily the determination of the level of calcium required to maintain balance in an adult simply estimates the individual's previous intake.

The report of the FAO-WHO Expert Group (*loc. cit.*) concludes that intakes of 400 to 500 mg. per day would represent the suggested practical allowance for adults, and asserts that the usefulness of an intake above this level has not been proven.

The adaptation shown by peoples eating low calcium diets is achieved by a more efficient absorption of dietary calcium than in persons accustomed to higher intakes. Adaptation to lower levels of calcium intake has been convincingly demonstrated in man (Malm, *loc. cit.*) and animals (K. M. Kon *et al.*, *Acta Biochim. Polon.* **7,** *167* (*1960*); S. N. Gershoff, M. A. Legg, and D. M. Hegsted, *J. Nutrition* **64,** *303* (*1958*)). J. M. Boda and H. H. Cole (*Ann. N.Y. Acad. Sci.* **64,** *370* (*1956*)) found that the occurrence of milk fever in lactating dairy cattle could in part be prevented by limiting the calcium intake somewhat prior to parturition. Presumably the mechanisms required to mobilize and efficiently utilize calcium are operative at the time of great need.

While the studies available demonstrate that man can adapt to lower levels of intake, they do not demonstrate that the lowest level studied is the minimal intake at which balance can be achieved, nor do they provide evidence that either the high or low level is most beneficial, detrimental, or immaterial.

In pregnancy, when bone is being formed, and during lactation, requirements for calcium are increased. Normal and prolonged lactation is not uncommon in women consuming relatively low levels of calcium, and one would expect that the normal adaptive mechanisms would respond to the greater need and dietary calcium would be more efficiently utilized. However, osteomalacia does develop in women after repeated pregnancies and lactations in some parts of the world. These cases apparently respond to vitamin D therapy even though dietary intake of calcium is not markedly increased.

Loss of bone usually begins about 45 years of age and may be an inevitable accompaniment of aging. It has been estimated that 14 million women in the United States alone have a significant degree of osteoporosis. Osteoporosis is common in other countries with relatively high calcium intakes, such as England and Scandinavia, but good data on prevalence are not available. There are practically no data from countries where the intake is habitually low. Although high calcium diets are recommended in the treatment of osteoporosis, the apparent calcium retentions observed in balance studies are not supported by the expected increases in bone density.

Recent evidence implicates fluoride deficiency as an important cause. The prevalence of osteoporosis is much lower in communities with high fluoride water supplies (over 4 p.p.m.) than in those with low fluoride water supplies (N. C. Leone *et al.*,

Arch. Indust. Health **21,** *324* (*1960*); D. S. Bernstein *et al., J. Am. Med. Assn.* **198,** *499* (*1966*)).

A number of clinical conditions are associated with evidence of excessive calcium in serum or urine, or calcification of the soft tissues: the idiopathic hypercalcemia of infancy, the "milk alkali syndrome," hypercalcuria, and kidney stones. High calcium intakes may be a contributing factor, since low calcium intakes are part of effective therapy, but epidemiologic data are not available to support this conclusion.

Deposition of radiostrontium in the skeleton is influenced by the ^{90}Sr/Ca ratio and the total calcium in the diet. It will tend to be high when the ratio is high and when the dietary intake of calcium is low relative to need. The relationships are rather complex and large changes in the diet may be required to produce relatively small changes in radiostrontium deposition. The practicality of such programs at times of high fallout remains to be demonstrated and must be evaluated against the possible detrimental effects.

Phosphorus

Phosphorus compounds play a central role in transformations of energy in the body, and an understanding of "high energy phosphate bonds" has been one of the major recent achievements in biochemistry. Adenosinetriphosphate and the nucleotides formed from several of the vitamins are essential in the catabolism and anabolism of carbohydrates, fats, and proteins. The nucleoproteins containing phosphorus make up a large portion of the nuclear material and also occur in the cytoplasm of all cells and are key materials in the processes of cell division, reproduction, and transmission of hereditary characteristics. The viruses which somehow modify normal cell function to reproduce themselves are also nucleoproteins. Among the fat soluble materials one finds a great variety of phospholipids. Numerous advances have been made in identification of these substances in recent years.

Blood and serum phosphorus is generally classified as lipid, ester, and inorganic. Inorganic phosphorus in infants' serum is between 5 and 6.6 mg. per 100 ml., and gradually diminishes to the adult level of 3 to 4 mg. Ordinarily there is a reverse relationship between the serum inorganic phosphate and serum calcium, but this is not always so.

It is likely that most, if not all, phosphorus is absorbed as free phosphorus. The various inorganic esters must thus be hydrolyzed, probably by the various phosphatases, prior to absorption. Absorption of inorganic phosphorus is in part related to the amount of calcium in the diet, or other similar materials which may form insoluble salts, and thus related to absorption of calcium as well. Iron, strontium, beryllium, and the like also form insoluble phosphates. As indicated above, the Ca/P ratio is probably of little significance in adult man.

Fecal phosphorus represents both unabsorbed phosphorus and that secreted into the tract. The amounts from the two sources are not well defined and absorption of both is presumably affected by the same factors. Under ordinary conditions the feces contain about 30 per cent of the amount in the diet. Dietary phosphorus is thus absorbed better than calcium and, consequently, kidney excretion of phosphorus is much greater than that of calcium.

Urinary phosphorus is largely inorganic phosphate, the amount depending primarily upon the amount absorbed from the intestinal tract. Oxidation of sugar requires phosphorus, and there is a temporary lowering of serum phosphates and of phosphate excretion after ingestion of carbohydrates. Catabolism of body tissues in starvation, acidosis, and the like, releases considerable phosphorus, which is excreted by the kidney.

Relatively few data are available on actual phosphorus requirements under different conditions. The Food and Nutrition Board (*Recommended Dietary Allowances, 1964*) has concluded that the allowances should at least equal those for calcium in diets of children and women during the latter part of pregnancy and lactation. For other adults they are said to be about 1.5 times those for calcium.

Magnesium

The adult body contains approximately 25 g. magnesium, and therefore it is one of the major mineral constituents. It is primarily an intracellular ion and adult fat free tissue contains about 43 mg. per kilogram. The serum level is approximately 2 mEq per liter. Although it has long been known that it is an essential nutrient for rats, data indicating a significant role for magnesium in practical human nutrition have only recently been presented. Analytical determination methods for magnesium have much improved, with the expected results. It is now known to be required for the activity of a great many enzymes, particularly those concerned with oxidative phosphorylation. Such functions do not yet explain the signs or symptoms observed in the nutritional deficiency (W. E. C. Wacker and B. L. Vallee, *New Engl. J. Med.* **259**, *431* (1958)).

Young rats fed diets devoid of magnesium develop within a few days a marked vasodilation, followed by necrotic changes and convulsive seizures which often result in death. Of particular interest is the observation that the calcification of many soft tissues which occurs in surviving animals can also be produced in animals fed diets only marginally deficient. The amounts of magnesium required to prevent lesions and deficiency signs are dependent on the amounts of calcium and phosphorus (and perhaps other nutrients) fed.

Rats and monkeys fed diets limiting in magnesium are considerably more susceptible to atherosclerosis induced by cholesterol feeding (J. J. Vitale *et al., Circ. Res.* **12**, *642* (1963)). Diets high in magnesium are partially effective in preventing deposition of oxalate stones in rats with oxaluria induced by feeding diets deficient in vitamin B_6 (S. N. Gershoff and S. B. Andrus, *J. Nutrition* **73**, *308* (1961)).

Clear cut evidence of magnesium deficiency in man has recently been described (Wacker, F. D. Moore, D. D. Ulmer, and Vallee, *J. Am. Med. Assn.* **180**, *161* (1962); R. D. Montgomery, *Lancet* **2**, *74* (1960)). Hypomagnesemic tetany, very similar to hypocalemic tetany, is distinguished by the serum calcium and magnesium levels and prompt response to magnesium administration. Recent evidence based upon adequate methodology leaves no doubt that magnesium deficiency may be a substantial clinical problem. There is no satisfactory evidence of the normal requirement, but values of 150 mg. per day for infants, 400 mg. per day during pregnancy and lactation, and 250 mg. per day for adults have been suggested as adequate.

Our thanks to the contributors to this booklet for giving so generously of their time and knowledge, and for their observation of our space requirements, which limited the number of words and references.

CONTRIBUTORS

WILLIAM B. BEAN, M.D.
University of Iowa, Iowa City

WILLIAM F. BRIDGERS, M.D.
University of Miami, Miami

W. DUANE BROWN, PH.D.
University of California, Berkeley

WILLIAM J. DARBY, M.D., PH.D.
Vanderbilt University, Nashville

HELEN M. DYER, PH.D.
Federation of American Societies for Experimental Biology, Bethesda

GILBERT B. FORBES, M.D.
University of Rochester, Rochester

WENDELL H. GRIFFITH, PH.D.
Federation of American Societies for Experimental Biology, Bethesda

W. STANLEY HARTROFT, M.D., PH.D.
The Hospital for Sick Children, Toronto

D. MARK HEGSTED, PH.D.
Harvard School of Public Health, Boston

ROBERT E. HODGES, M.D.
University of Iowa, Iowa City

WILLIAM G. HOEKSTRA, PH.D.
University of Wisconsin, Madison

OGDEN C. JOHNSON, PH.D.
National Institutes of Health, Bethesda

RICHARD J. JONES, M.D.
University of Chicago, Chicago

C. GLEN KING, PH.D.
St. Luke's Hospital Center, New York

MICHAEL C. LATHAM, M.B., M.P.H., D.T.M. & H.
Harvard School of Public Health, Boston

ORVILLE A. LEVANDER, PH.D.
Food and Drug Administration, Washington, D. C.

STANLEY LEVEY, PH.D.
University Hospitals of Cleveland, Cleveland

JAMES F. MEAD, PH.D.
University of California, Los Angeles

OLAF MICKELSEN, PH.D.
Michigan State University, East Lansing

ROBERT E. OLSON, M.D., PH.D.
St. Louis University, St. Louis

JAMES C. PEDEN, JR., M.D.
Washington University, St. Louis

EDUARDO A. PORTA, M.D.
Hospital for Sick Children, Toronto

OSWALD A. ROELS, PH.D.
Columbia University, Palisades, N.Y.

HAROLD H. SANDSTEAD, M.D.
Vanderbilt University, Nashville

JAMES H. SHAW, PH.D.
Harvard School of Dental Medicine, Boston

JOSEPH J. VITALE, PH.D.
Tufts University College of Medicine, Boston

MARY ANN WILLIAMS, PH.D.
University of California, Berkeley